Smart Surgeons
Sharp Decisions

Cognitive skills
to avoid errors & achieve results

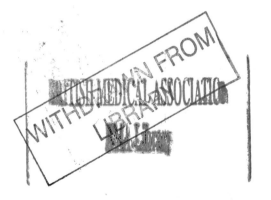

Uttam Shiralkar MS FRCS MRCPsych

The Surgical Psychology Series

tfm Publishing Limited, Castle Hill Barns, Harley, Nr Shrewsbury, SY5 6LX, UK.
Tel: +44 (0)1952 510061; Fax: +44 (0)1952 510192
E-mail: nikki@tfmpublishing.com; Web site: www.tfmpublishing.com

Design & Typesetting: Nikki Bramhill BSc Hons Dip Law
First Edition: © January 2011
ISBN: 978 1 903378 81 6

Printed by Gutenberg Press Ltd., Gudja Road, Tarxien, PLA 19, Malta.
Tel: +356 21897037; Fax: +356 21800069.

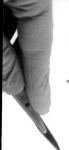

Contents

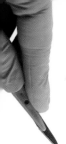

About the author

Uttam Shiralkar qualified and worked as a surgeon for 15 years in the USA, UK and India, before he decided to enter the field of psychological medicine. His new found interest in the budding field of psycho-oncology and the medical problems he faced after a car accident, were amongst the few reasons behind this move. While pursuing a career in psycho-oncology, it struck him strongly, how much of an impact a surgeon's psychology has on his/her clinical outcome. When he started sharing new research findings on this subject with surgical colleagues, they expressed a strong desire to learn more about it. What started as an informal chat with surgical colleagues became a day-long course 'Ergonomics for surgeons'. Currently, in addition to fulfilling his commitment as a consultant in the NHS, Uttam, on an informal level, is actively involved in mentoring surgeons at various levels of their careers. He lives in the West Midlands, with his son and wife, a Consultant Vascular Surgeon. (Interest disclosure: NO, he does not offer any therapy to his surgeon wife!)

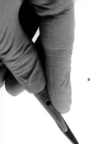

Foreword

I recall many years ago being impressed by an article in a Sunday newspaper entitled something like 'you can teach monkeys to be surgeons'. Scientists had managed to get chimps to learn certain technical aspects of a surgical procedure. The authors of the article speculated whether in the future primates might be able to take on simple, standard surgical procedures. And all this was years ago, long before the surgical robot had been thought of! The fundamental misconception, that surgery is only a technical skill, remains hard to shake off, particularly with the advent of single procedure practitioners such as nurse endoscopists and hernia nurse practitioners.

Patients prefer to think that surgeons, like robots, always work at the peak of performance, consistently at the top of their game. No-one imagines a surgeon can have an off day, be in a bad mood, feel unwell, or be just plain bored. Here's the shocker: surgeons are human too!

So anyone who wants to be a smart surgeon has to know more than just anatomy and physiology. The smart surgeon has to have insight into how their feelings and behaviour can alter performance. They must understand their own limitations, and be able to manage themselves through good days and bad, through success and failure, and deal professionally with patients who may be unfairly disgruntled or even surprisingly satisfied. In short they need the insight to be able to step back and evaluate themselves.

This book is first about understanding that there is a great deal to being a surgeon more than knowledge alone; it is a framework to help an individual to get the best out of themselves every day through triumph and adversity. We watch Formula 1 racing drivers try to squeeze extra seconds of performance out of their cars, because that is the difference between winning and losing a race. Squeezing that extra bit of individual performance is the difference between being a good surgeon and a great one.

This book is not for monkeys; it is for the surgeon who wishes to be more than a good technician, one who can optimise their own performance and behaviour with insight and intelligence.

Jonothan J Earnshaw DM FRCS
Consultant Vascular Surgeon
Gloucestershire Royal Hospital
Gloucester, UK
Editor-in-Chief, *British Journal of Surgery*

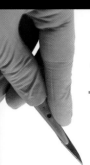

Acknowledgements

Firstly, I would like to acknowledge the support of Dr Ros Keeton, Chief Executive of the Worcestershire Mental Health Partnership Trust in starting the 'Ergonomics for Surgeons' course. I would also like to thank my friend and colleague, Phil Higton, with whom I ran this course. We are aiming to roll out several courses in the near future covering the subject matter within this book.

I would also like to acknowledge many of my colleagues from a range of surgical specialties who supported this novel idea and have in many different ways contributed to this book, especially Mr Tony Giddings, Mr John Watkinson and Mr Martin Portman who all gave valuable feedback after reading the manuscript.

Thanks go to all the publishers and authors who have given permission to use the excerpts from their books. Special thanks goes to Mr Buzz Reed who handled the permission matter on behalf of Klein Associates and Robert Hamm who kindly allowed me to use the material without any restrictions.

I am especially indebted to my friend, Dr Ponkshe, who provided the photographs for the cover and other images in the book. Others who I would like to thank are Penny Billingham in preparing the manuscript, Jenny Murray for organizing the course at the Charles Hasting Centre, and Dr Sanjay Suri for giving valuable comments while preparing the manuscript.

And finally, I would like to thank Nikki Bramhill, Director of tfm publishing, for being proactive and considerate throughout the process of creation of this book. This being my first endeavour, it would have been difficult without Nikki's expertise and interest in this subject. Whilst working with Nikki, it felt that writing a book is very easy – I can do it many more times!

We gratefully acknowledge the permission granted to reuse material from the following:

1. Chapter 3: p19-21, 23, 24

Groopman J. Surgery and satisfaction. *How Doctors Think.*

Reproduced with permission from Dr Jerome Groopman MD, © 2007 Dr Jerome Groopman, and the following publishers: Houghton Mifflin Harcourt Publishing Company, New York, USA; All rights reserved (www.hmhbooks.com); Byword Books Private Limited, Delhi, India (www.bywordbooks.in); Scribe Publications, Carlton North, VIC, Australia (www.scribepublications.com.au).

2. Chapter 5: p88

Finkelstein S, Whitehead J, Campbell A. *Think Again: Why Good Leaders Make Bad Decisions and How to Keep It From Happening to You.* Harvard Business Press, 2009.

Reproduced with permission from Harvard Business Publishing.

3. Chapter 5: p67-69, p76-78, p81; Chapter 7 p107, p114-5.

Klein G. *Sources of Power.* MIT Press, 1998.
Klein G. *Power of Intuition.* MIT Press, 1998.

Reproduced with permission from Klein Associates, Division of Applied Research Associates, Inc., USA.

4. Chapter 6

Abernathy CM, Hamm RM. *Surgical Scripts.* Hanley & Belfus Inc., 1994.

Reproduced with permission from Dr Hamm and Elsevier Inc.

We also acknowledge permission to reuse the following illustrations:

1. Images on p1, p3, p11, p14, p15, p19, p31, p35, p40, p41, p46, p48, p54, p55, p57, p58, p62, p63, p65, p67, p76, p78, p81, p91, p107, p114, p119, p120, p123, p131, p133.

Reproduced with permission from Shutterstock Images LLC.

2. p5 WHO Surgical Safety Checklist.

Reproduced with permission from http://www.who.int/patientsafety/safesurgery/ss_checklist/en/index.html.

3. Images on p8, p19, p91, p110

Reproduced with permission from Image 100 Ltd, © 1999.

4. p88 Checker shadow.

Reproduced with permission from http://web.mit.edu/persci/people/adelson/checkershadow_illusion.htm.

5. Images on p111, p115

Klein G. *Power of Intuition*. MIT Press, 1998.

Reproduced with permission from Klein Associates Division of Applied Research Associates, Inc., USA.

6. p107 ultrasound image. Mernagh JR, Mohide PT, Lappalainen RE, Fedoryshin JG. US assessment of the fetal head and neck: a state-of-the-art pictoral review. *RadioGraphics* 1999; 19: S229-41.

Reproduced with permission from the Radiological Society of North America, © 1999.

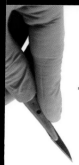

Dedication

Behind every successful man stands a woman
telling him that he is wrong

For me (successful…?), it has not been just one, but two women!

I dedicate this book to both of them,
my mother and wife.

I also dedicate this book to my son, Saarth.

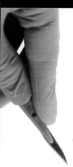

Introduction

Before the incision is made

The idea for this book came to me while I was running a course called 'Ergonomics for Surgeons' with my colleague from aviation, Phil Higton. The purpose of the course was to highlight the importance of non-technical skills in surgery. Having worked in surgery for over 15 years, I was conscious that we do not pay much attention to these 'soft skills'. Like every other surgeon, I was not mindful of them until I started working in psychological medicine. When I realised the value of these skills, I felt that if I had known about these skills while I was training in surgery or when I was practising as a surgeon, my performance would have significantly benefited. I wanted to share this knowledge with my surgical colleagues through the course. I was very pleased with the feedback I received from surgeons who attended the course. Later, some of them reported a positive impact on their performance as well. Their encouraging responses motivated me to take the decision of taking a step further.

I was curious about how surgeons would respond to the endeavour of writing a book on this unusual topic. I gave the manuscript to my surgical colleagues in order to get their feedback. I was delighted to hear that they had not come across a book on this topic before: "It is unique," they told me. Obviously, I was pleased with these comments. However, I thought "this was an interesting paradox." Although this book may be unique, the contents are common: common in the sense that they are about your day-to-day professional activity; common in the sense that they are applicable to all surgical specialties; and common in the sense that they are useful for anybody, irrespective of seniority. A senior surgeon wrote to me and said, "I don't know how I survived this far without knowing all this." The information provided here is so common or, to be more precise, so fundamental – that we take it for granted. We are expected to know all that is described here, but hardly anybody bothers to explain it to us. While preparing this book, I realised why we are not being told about these things: because they are difficult to explain. While reading this book, you may think, at times, "I know all of this." In that case, ask yourself, "Would I be able to explain it to somebody else?" I bet the answer would be: "Yes, but it is very difficult." I have attempted to simplify this complex subject into a simple and clinically relevant format.

During my career in surgery, I had the opportunity to observe and work with some exceptionally smart surgeons. I have been in the habit of analysing the reasons behind their extraordinary performance and trying to find out why others can't match them. Over the years, I gained some understanding of these questions from cognitive science. This book is my attempt to 'cherry pick' some of those facts that are important to every surgeon.

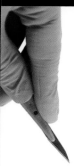

Chapter 1

Checkmate – the checklist phenomenon

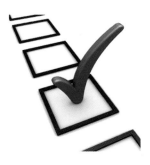

In February 2006, I was invited to participate in a course to train surgeons in 'non-technical skills'. The other invitees, numbering about fifteen, were senior consultant surgeons from a range of specialties.

At the start of the course, we were asked to watch a video of eight basketball players – half dressed in black and half in white – passing the ball to each other. The facilitator asked us to watch the clip carefully and to count the number of passes that the team in white made. The video lasted for only 2-3 minutes.

When the video ended, the facilitator asked, "How many passes did you see the team in white make?"

"Thirteen," was our confident reply.

Without confirming whether this was the correct number of passes or not, the facilitator asked, "Did you see anything else in the video, apart from the players making the passes?"

None of us had.

"Are you sure that none of you noticed anything besides the players?"

Nobody responded to this question, as we didn't want to appear to be foolish, in case we had missed something important.

"Didn't you see a gorilla?" asked the facilitator.

"What? A gorilla?" We laughed, thinking that it must be some kind of joke.

"Yes," said the facilitator, "there was a gorilla in the video. Didn't you see it?"

We were a bit perplexed, and said, "No," with a hint of disbelief.

"Now watch the clip again, this time without counting the passes," said the facilitator.

When we watched the clip for the second time, everybody went quiet a few seconds after the clip had started. We saw a person wearing a gorilla suit enter from one corner. The gorilla walked to the centre, where players were making passes, stood there waving its hands, and then left the scene at the other corner, having been on screen for nearly ten seconds.

We were stunned when we saw the video again. We could not believe that we had missed such an obvious thing! One of the group said, "We surgeons consider ourselves good at picking up visual cues. This experiment shatters that belief!" It wasn't the case that the gorilla was small and camouflaged against the players – in fact, it was quite prominent and hard to ignore, even for a casual observer. Still, us 'careful observers' had missed it.

It may be difficult to appreciate the experience of watching the video and the feeling of disbelief of missing the gorilla just by reading this description. If you are interested in watching this video, it is available on YouTube. Transport for London has adapted the experiment to educate the public about traffic awareness; it is available on http://www.dothetest.co.uk/. We think that we notice far more of the world around us than we actually do. Car drivers who crash into motorcycles often state that they did not see them, or that the motorcycle came out of nowhere, because they're expecting and looking out for cars and not motorcycles.

The experiment on the surgical course was intended to make surgeons aware of the limitations of their powers of observation, however clever they may be. It was also intended to highlight the fact that, when we attend to a specific task, we overlook things that are out of range due to limited observation spans. The problem is that we are not aware that we are unable to see the whole picture. Until we come across situations like the 'gorilla' experiment, we assume that we see whatever is needed to be seen. We do not question surgeons' abilities in these kinds of basic tasks. Obviously, these experiences challenge your views.

I have seen this video being shown to other groups of surgeons, and the results are the same every time. The more I observe surgeons watching the video, the more I see the wider implications of this experiment. The gorilla represents many other things that surgeons fail to notice. I realised that, on a broader scale, surgeons have focused their attention on counting the numbers (of passes), as in making technological advances but, have overlooked the 'human factors' in day to day practice (the gorilla). The gorilla symbolises all the non-technical aspects of surgical practice that surgeons take for granted – such as, as in this case, a surgeon's cognitive skills. For all the astonishing surgical know-how we have accumulated, failures are still frequent in surgical practice. One of the reasons is increasingly evident – the volume and complexity of what is known exceeds the capacity of surgeons to deliver it. This is due to a lack of focus on human factors, at a systemic and individual level. The complexity of surgical practice has now overwhelmed the ability of an individual's brain to manage it, however expert and specialised he may be. As a result, basic steps are sometimes missed, which are a matter of life and death for patients.

There is a reason to mention the gorilla experiment here. It is to do with the hullabaloo surrounding the WHO surgical checklist. If you look at the 'surgical

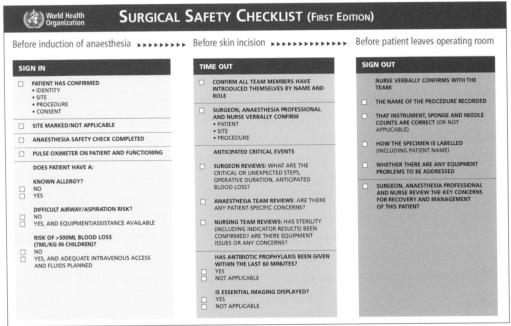

THIS CHECKLIST IS NOT INTENDED TO BE COMPREHENSIVE. ADDITIONS AND MODIFICATIONS TO FIT LOCAL PRACTICE ARE ENCOURAGED.

Reproduced with permission from http://www.who.int/patientsafety/safesurgery/ss_checklist/en/index.html.

checklist' as a tool to help us spot the 'gorilla' in operating theatres, you can see the correlation between the gorilla experiment and the checklist. There are some differences between the gorilla in the video and the gorillas in the operating theatres, however. At least the gorilla that you see in the video is harmless. It just stands in the centre, trying to show its presence. It neither disturbs the game nor bothers the players. However, the 'gorillas' in operating theatres are not necessarily benign. They don't just stand by and let you do your business without disturbing you. They can create problems for us, and they do. They affect us – they have an impact on surgical outcomes, and yet still we fail to notice them, thinking that they are irrelevant. We remain busy counting passes, unaware that the gorilla may be disturbing the game. The checklist is supposed to spot the gorilla in the operating theatre before it creates any problems.

From the start of 2010, use of the surgical checklist has become mandatory in England and Wales. However, very few surgeons have been enthusiastic about its implementation. It has been in the news with conflicting comments. Some have described it as the biggest clinical innovation in the past 30 years, while others have dismissed it as just another 'tick-box exercise', favoured by hospital management who are keen to get mortality and morbidity figures down by the cheapest available means. Some have gone further in saying that these cheap ways of improving the results of surgery are an insult to the profession, while others have hailed the checklist as one of the greatest discoveries in the history of surgery, possibly even eclipsing the introduction of antisepsis, asepsis and antibiotics [1]. Having come across such diverse opinions, I decided to gather more information about the checklist project.

The surgical-checklist project was sponsored by the World Health Organization (WHO). An international consultative process produced a nineteen-item surgical checklist which takes no longer than two minutes to apply [2]. The checklist is supposed to be applied at three points: during the pre-operative check-in phase; in the operating room prior to the surgical incision; and after the completion of the operation. The study involved eight centres from five continents and included places as diverse as teaching hospitals in North America and a rural hospital in Africa. St Mary's Hospital in London was the pilot site in the UK. Lord Darzi was actively involved at a national, as well as international level, in this project. The study prospectively enrolled 7,688 adult patients undergoing surgery: 3,733 before the implementation of the checklist and 3,955 afterwards. The endpoints were compared for these two time periods.

Wondering why the WHO got involved in this venture, I became aware that, according to the WHO, the annual volume of major surgery was estimated at 234 million operations per year all over the world. Surgical deaths and complications have become a global public-health problem. Even in industrialised countries, the rate of complications from surgery ranges from 3-17%. To give you an example, in the United States, the state of Minnesota, which has less than 2% of the US population, reported 21 wrong-site surgeries in a single year. Remember, this is the reported incidence of an event that should never happen in the developed world. The real situation is probably even worse, because most critical incidents like these are not reported. According to the WHO, surgical complications contribute to approximately one million deaths around the world each year. As far as the situation in the UK is concerned, more than eight million patients undergo surgical procedures every year, equivalent to one in every eight people. In 2007 alone, 129,419 untoward surgical incidences were reported to the National Patient Safety Agency (NPSA) [3]. Over 1,000 incidences resulted in severe harm and 271 led to the death of the patient. The WHO estimates that, each year, half a million – in other words, 50% – of the deaths related to surgery are preventable. Thus, as part of a global "Safe Surgery Saves Lives" programme, the WHO developed a simple, short checklist of guidelines for safe surgical procedures.

The study, published in the *New England Journal of Medicine* [4], showed that use of the checklist reduced the rate of major complications by 36% (from 11% to 7%, p<0.001), deaths by 47% (from 1.5% to 0.8%, p=0.003), and infections by almost half. The reduction in deaths and complications was similar across all the hospitals in the study. The results were startling! If indeed 234 million surgical procedures are performed annually, and the average percentage of deaths can be reduced by 0.7%, that would mean that 1,638,000 lives could be saved worldwide and disabilities reduced by another few million. This too by using a method that takes just 90 seconds to use and it is free of charge!

If you are thinking that these results are too good to be true, you are not alone. Even the researchers did not expect such a profound effect [5]. They acknowledged that part of the improvement might result from the Hawthorne effect – an improvement in performance just because the individual is aware that he/she is being observed [6]. Sometimes people perform better when they are participants in an experiment. These individuals change their behaviour purely because of the attention they receive for a limited period. That being said, however, the Hawthorne effect is unlikely to have played a significant role in the case of the checklist. Since half of the participant surgeons were not keen about the use of the checklist at the start of the project, why would they bother to change their behaviour to please researchers who did not interest them? Dr Gawande, a lead researcher, revealed that he met significant resistance from participating surgeons, especially during the initial period of the study. About half of the surgeons said that the checklist made sense; of the other half, 30% were unenthusiastic but complied, while the remaining 20% said that they thought it was a waste of time and declined the invitation to participate. Although some surgeons refused to use the checklist initially, they became aware that the results were improving as they went along. By the end, only about 20% of surgeons said they didn't like the checklist; interestingly, though, 93% said that they would want it used if they were undergoing an operation themselves! Let's be honest – we don't like checklists. They can be laborious. They're not much fun. Some may see a checklist as an irritation and an incursion on their terrain. For others, the lack of enthusiasm is most likely an expression of a belief that the process is little more than a distraction. It is understandable that there will be resistance to adopting something as mundane as a checklist. Early adopters will already be using them. Some will be convinced by the research evidence, while others will want data from their own practice. But a few will see checklists as an insult to their professionalism and will never be convinced.

We are missing an important point (again, a gorilla point!) in the midst of these different opinions about the merits and demerits of the checklist and the appropriateness of the results of the study. The important point is, a simple intervention to change a practice behaviour can make a big impact on surgical outcome. What the checklist did was to bring about a change in the behaviour of the operating team. It changed what is known as 'team cognition' – in other words, the collective thinking of the entire team. You can imagine that if such a transient change in the

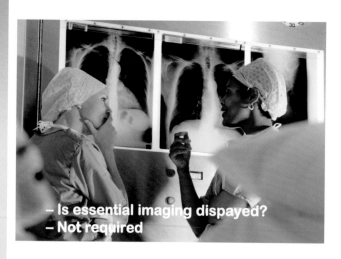

– Is essential imaging dispayed?
– Not required

behaviour of the surgical team could have so significant impact, what would happen if the behaviour changed for a sustained period? We might assume that the change in behaviour of the operating team members was due to the Hawthorne effect, but why should we not then think about creating a consistent Hawthorne effect? While we are occupied in discussing whether to use the checklist and, if so, how to use it (counting the passes), we are closing our eyes to the reality that, while managing surgical patients, we may fail to notice some basic things (gorilla), and yet by making some cognitive changes, we can spot the gorilla and improve our performance. In other words, surgeons can correctly count the passes as well as keep an eye on the gorilla.

This is not just about the checklist and the surgical team; it is also about you, an individual surgeon. The manner in which the behavioural change of the team improved the surgical outcome; it can also be seen in individual surgeons. It seems that some surgeons are able to create a 'checklist' in their heads. In the same way that the WHO checklist affected the team's cognition, the checklist in the surgeon's head affects his thinking. You would agree that not all surgeons function equally effectively. Some are better organised than others. Some spot problems sooner than others. What creates these differences? The answer is the checklist in their heads. Cognitive science calls it a 'pattern', and refers to the process of using the checklist as 'pattern recognition'.

In a sense, the WHO checklist has modified a natural process of pattern recognition for the purpose of team functioning. It is more systematic – as some surgeons are. It has clarity – as some surgeons have. And it has been effective – as some...! To be honest, this is not the first time that a checklist has been used in operating theatres, as nurses have been using one for some time. This is not the first time that it has been shown to be effective for clinical outcomes, as Peter Pronovast in the USA has shown on the efficacy of a checklist for nosocomial infections. Medical professionals are not the first ones to try it; pilots have been using checklists for decades. So, what is exciting about this surgical checklist in particular? One of the exciting things is the way it has applied the principles of cognitive science. The cognitive limitation that causes us to miss the gorilla in the video has been turned on its head, and a restructuring of cognitive processes has been achieved.

To make a final comment, I would use an analogy from chess. The introduction of the checklist should not be seen as checkmate – in other words, as the end of the problems in operating theatres – but instead surgeons would be benefited if they adopt a friendly approach or become a mate with the principles behind the checklist. The principles behind the checklist are the principles of cognitive science. As the gorilla experiment and the checklist study have shown, let's not just count the passes and check the boxes; watch out for gorillas and think about the human factors in surgical practice.

Key points

- Due to the limitations of our sensory system, surgeons are unable to pick up all the relevant information related to their tasks.

- The price that we pay for these limitations is very high in surgical practice worldwide.

- Surgeons need to be aware of these limitations and the methods that can be used to compensate for these problems.

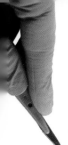

Chapter 2

To err is surgeon – human factors in surgery

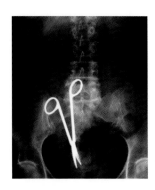

The Institute of Medicine, an influential organisation in the USA, published a report in 1999 entitled *To Err is Human*. It reported the gravity of hospital errors in the USA. Among other things, they reported that 20,000 people die in the USA every year after elective surgeries [7]. These are the mortality figures; morbidity figures are not mentioned. We have to keep in mind that these figures are for elective surgeries. As we know, the rate of complications is higher for emergency procedures. If we extrapolate these mortality figures to air travel, they would be the equivalent of two jumbo jets crashing every week, killing all the passengers. If that was the current state of air travel, how comfortable would you be while flying with your family? After the report was published, The *New York Times* wrote that if an airline had disclosed this kind of safety record, it would have been out of business overnight!

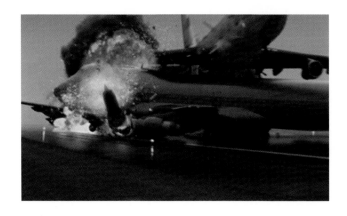

Consider for example the infamous 1977 Tenerife disaster, the deadliest accident in aviation history [8]. In March 1977, two Boeing 747s collided on the runway at Tenerife airport. Both planes were prepared for departure from the airport. One of the planes was a KLM plane and the other one was Pan Am. The KLM plane was waiting for air traffic control clearance. The Pan Am plane was instructed to taxi onto the runway and then to exit onto another taxi way. The KLM plane was given air traffic control clearance for the route it was to fly – but not clearance to begin take-off. The KLM captain apparently mistook this message for take-off clearance. He proceeded to accelerate his plane down the runway. Due to the fog, the KLM crew did not see the Pan Am taxiing ahead of them. The jets could not be seen by the control tower. In total 583 people died!

Let's see how things have changed since that incident.

In 2009, a US Airways flight took off from New York with 155 people on board. Immediately after take-off, it struck a large flock of Canadian geese and both engines shut down. It is not unusual for planes to hit birds, but a dual bird strike is rare. Jet engines are designed to cope with most birds by liquifying them. However, because Canadian geese are large, the engines shut down. Once the captain realised that both engines had failed, he took control of the plane and made an instinctive decision to do a crash landing in the Hudson River. All the passengers survived. Captain Sullenberger was hailed as a hero. But as details later revealed of the procedures and checklists involved, the co-pilot who shared flight responsibilities, and the cabin crew who handled the swift evacuation, people started to wonder about exactly who the hero was. As the captain himself acknowledged, the outcome was the result of teamwork and adherence to the checklist as much as the instinctive decisions he had made.

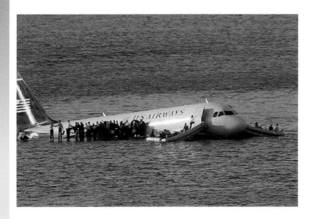

If you are wondering how these two opposite outcomes in aviation can be explained, the answer is the acknowledgement of a human factor. The aviation industry had been analysing accidents for several decades and found that 73% of accidents were due to human factors: problems relating to communication, team co-ordination and decision-making. The way in which individuals perform within systems is referred to as the human factor, a concept that arose during investigations into calamities in air transport and nuclear power plants – that is, in organisations where safety depends upon a high degree of reliability. Aviation has taken all these findings seriously and has made appropriate changes at an organisational as well as an individual level.

The question is: can the airline-safety model work in surgery? Surgery and aviation have important similarities. Pilots and surgeons are highly trained professionals who operate in complex environments, where teams interact with technology. In both domains, risk varies from low to high, with threats coming from a variety of sources. Safety is a paramount goal for both professions. The medical venues where parallels with aviation have been explored most fully are the operating rooms. Helmreich and Merritt have examined aspects of the professional cultures of pilots and of doctors working in the operating room, anaesthetists, and surgeons [9]. They found both positive and negative similarities between the cultures. Positively speaking, both groups are proud of being members of an elite professional group that requires extensive training and selective qualification. On the negative side, both pilots and doctors tend to deny personal vulnerability, believing that their decision-making is as good in emergencies as under normal conditions.

Human-factor science – which is also known as 'Ergonomics', a trendier label – has developed over the years and has formed subspecialties. One of the subspecialties is physical ergonomics. In the case of surgery, this subspecialty deals with the design of surgical equipment. For example, physical ergonomics has played a role in the design of operating microscopes, surgical endoscopes, and surgical robotics. The second subspecialty is organisational ergonomics. And the third subspecialty is cognitive ergonomics, which is of our main interest. It deals with judgement, decision-making and other thought processes involved in day-to-day work.

If you are unfamiliar with the concept of human-factor science, you might think that it may not have a significant clinical application. Would you accept its clinical importance given that, after studying 1,440,776 critical events in operating theatres, investigators reported that human factors were responsible for 54% of cardiac arrests, 74% of other critical events, and 71% of deaths among those patients? [10] When adverse events in operating theatres were analysed, it was found that many of the incidences occurred not because of a lack of technical expertise, but because of failure of non-technical – in other words, human factors [11]. One shouldn't comfort oneself by thinking that problems occur because of inexperience or in unusual cases. When Thomas Hugh reviewed 133 surgical malpractice claims, it revealed that the majority of errors (73%) involved experienced surgeons, and in 84% of the cases the procedure was 'routine' [12]. Among all the adverse events in any hospital, around 40-50% occurs in the operating theatre [13], and 27% of claims against a hospital are due to cognitive errors in theatre [14]. An element as simple as communication was a causal factor in 43% of errors made in surgery [15].

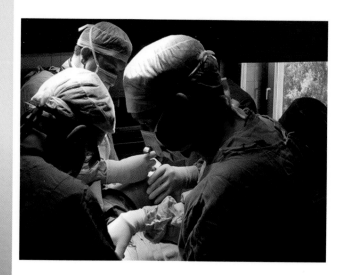

Alfred Cuschieri suggests that, "The propensity for error is so intrinsic to human behaviour that scientifically it is best considered as inherently biologic, since faultless performance and error results from the same mental process" [13]. Error is the flip-side of correct human performance, and is itself the product of cognitive ability and level of psychomotor skill, which in professions requiring dexterity and hand-eye co-ordination (such as surgery) determines safe and optimal execution (proficiency). The way we respond to surgical errors is interesting. On one hand, there are newsworthy or 'limelight' errors that hit the headlines and account for the majority of litigations, for example, wrong-side surgery and leaving instruments inside patients. On the other hand, there are 'Cinderella' errors like a resuscitation or prophylaxis error and situation awareness, which in the context of patient safety are probably more important because of their greater frequency. The problem lies in the fact that corrective measures are used against limelight errors, while defence systems against Cinderella errors are practically non-existent. We have not done much about 'gorillas', the cognitive errors.

What can surgeons do right now to begin to reduce these types of surgical errors? The best answer to this question comes courtesy of Winston Churchill. During World War II, Churchill made a colossal error when he failed to realise how vulnerable Singapore was to attack by a Japanese land invasion. This error led to Singapore's downfall. In Churchill's equivalent of a morbidity and mortality (M&M) review after Singapore's collapse, he asked four questions:

- Why didn't I know?

- Why wasn't I told?

- Why didn't I ask?

- Why didn't I tell what I knew? [16]

When things go wrong, it is usually because a series of failures has conspired to produce disaster. The M&M rounds should take this into account. Unfortunately, it does not always happen that way. For that reason, many experts see M&M meetings as an unhelpful approach to analysing error and improving performance in surgery. It is not enough to ask what a surgeon could do or should have done differently, so that he and others may learn from it for next time. The surgeon is sometimes the final actor in a chain of events that set him or her up to fail.

As Dr Gawande writes in his book, *Complications: A Surgeon's Notes On An Imperfect Science* [17], if errors were due to a subset of dangerous surgeons, you might expect malpractice cases or complaints to be concentrated among a small group of surgeons, but in fact they follow a uniform bell-shaped distribution. Most surgeons are sued or face an enquiry at least once in the course of their careers. Studies of specific types of error have found that repeat offenders are not the problem. The fact is that virtually everyone who cares for surgical patients will make a mistake or commit an act of negligence every couple of years. For this reason, we are seldom outraged when the press reports yet another surgical horror story. We usually have a different reaction: that could be me! The important question is not how to keep bad surgeons from harming patients, but how to keep good doctors from harming patients.

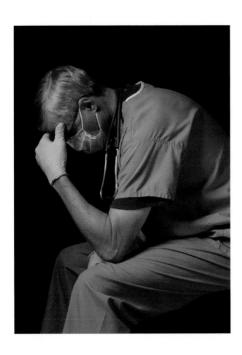

After they experience an untoward incident, some surgeons take negative reaction too far. It is one thing to be aware of one's limitations, but another to be infected by serious self-doubt. One surgeon experienced a case in which his patient suffered massive intra-abdominal bleeding and died on the operating table. Afterwards, the surgeon became reluctant to operate for months. When he did operate, he became indecisive. The case affected his performance for a long time. Even worse than losing self-confidence, however, is reacting defensively. There are surgeons who will see faults everywhere, except in themselves. They have no questions and no fears about their abilities. As a result, they learn nothing from their mistakes.

In the last few years, the 'systems' approach is dominant in the literature. Although systems are important, concentrating on those factors would not provide the entire solution, especially in surgery. We can make improvements by going after the system. But there are limitations to this emphasis on systems. It would be wrong for us, the individual performers, to give up our responsibility and our belief in perfection. The statistics may say that someday you will make a surgical error while operating, but each time when you are operating, you have to believe that with enough effort you can beat the odds. This isn't just professional pride: it is a necessary part of good surgical performance. This explains why concentrating on a 'system' is not enough. If you recollect an incident you may have encountered regarding surgical error, you would agree that various factors may have played their part, but it is ultimately you who was responsible for your actions. And also, changing the system may not be under your control, but changing your own behaviour is.

We cannot remedy problems that we don't know exist. There is reasonable evidence that clinicians fall short in noticing errors, making sense of them as events to be taken seriously. The quality of M&M meetings differs significantly. They are not seen by many as important and powerful educational tools. In a study [7], less than half of those who attended the meetings regularly (43% of trainees and 47% of consultants) found the meetings unhelpful, and gave low rankings for their "value in reducing error and improving care". The picture is one of half-hearted inquiries that are unlikely to spot errors and even less likely to spot remedies.

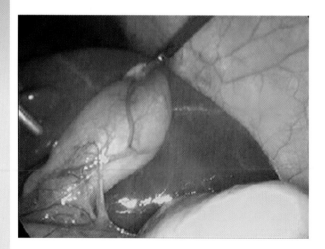

Bile duct injury is an indicator of avoidable surgical errors and cognitive factors. Removing the gallbladder is fairly straightforward, but there is a risk of cutting the bile duct; the mortality rate from bile duct injuries is significant. People think that it is purely a technical issue and that, if you have good surgical hands, you don't need to worry about this problem.

Studies show a different picture. Bile duct injury is an important unsolved problem of laparoscopic cholecystectomy, occurring with unacceptable frequency even in the hands of experienced surgeons. This suggests that a systemic predisposition to the injury is intrinsic to cholecystectomy and indicates that an analysis of the psychology and heuristics of surgical decision-making in relation to duct identification may be a guide to prevention. Errors leading to laparoscopic bile duct injuries stemmed principally from misperception, not errors of skill. The misperception was so compelling that in most cases the surgeon did not recognise the problem. Even when irregularities were identified, corrective feedback did not occur. These findings illustrate the complexity of human error in surgery [18]. Surgeons have found cognitive pills for these kinds of cognitive ills. Thomas Hugh, in a paper entitled 'New strategies to prevent laparoscopic bile duct injuries – surgeons can learn from pilots' [19], showed how cognitive techniques derived from aviation have reduced the incidence of bile duct injuries. These principles have been applied in a prospective study of 2,000 cases. The misidentification of biliary anatomy was the major cause of bile duct injuries and the injury remained unrecognised by the surgeon in 75% of cases, suggesting that traditional surgical teaching provides inadequate reference points to prevent duct misidentification and that spatial disorientation, analogous to navigation error, occurs. After human factors – educational principles derived from aviation crew resource management training – were applied, no bile duct injuries occurred in 2,000 cases.

The lesson we need take from these observations is, we need to go beyond conventional thinking to improve surgical performance. Cognitive skill like decision- making is one of them. The Australian surgeon, J Hall, in an article 'Cognition and surgeon' has suggested that surgeons have avoided looking inside their cognitive processes, just as tightrope walkers avoid looking at their feet for fear of falling [20]. However, a surgical career does not need to be a tightrope walk for the length of one's professional life. It should be a stroll. It is a good idea for a surgeon to see what is beneath his feet; so why not take a look at what goes on in your head while you are managing a surgical patient?

Key points

◆   Human factors play a crucial role in surgical mishaps or errors. Most of these incidences are preventable.

◆   Just as the manner in which aviation has taken human factors seriously and thus improved passenger safety, surgeons also need to acknowledge the impact of human factors on surgical outcome.

◆   Addressing cognitive factors will reduce the incidence of human factor errors.

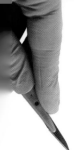

Chapter 3

Why good surgeons make bad decisions

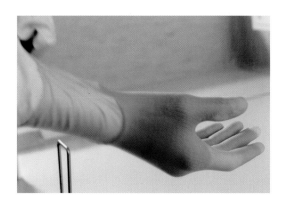

Dr Jerome Groopman, Chair of Medicine at the Harvard Medical School, had been troubled by pain and swelling in his right hand for a few months. When the symptoms did not resolve after several courses of medication, he consulted a hand surgeon – for the sake of confidentiality, let's call him Dr A. After the clinical examination and X-rays, Dr A could not find any abnormality apart from cysts in the scaphoid and lunate which, according to him, were not related to the problem. He advised Dr Groopman to use a splint for a month. Despite using the splint, the symptoms persisted, and an MRI scan was carried out. Even this did not reveal any pathology apart from the cysts. Over the course of the following year, Dr Groopman had various other investigations, tried splinting again and had local steroid injections. Nothing seemed to be working. Whenever Dr Groopman asked what was wrong with his wrist, Dr A would shrug his shoulders, expressing his inability to provide a diagnosis. After undergoing treatment for a year without any benefit, Dr Groopman expressed his concerns, to which Dr A replied that Dr Groopman had developed a "hyper-reactive synovium" and needed a surgery.

Not impressed by this unusual diagnosis and unclear treatment, Dr Groopman went to another orthopaedic surgeon – Dr B. At the outset, Dr B dismissed Dr A's diagnosis of a "hyper-reactive synovium" by remarking that such a term doesn't exist. When Dr B saw the X-rays and MRI he found not just the cysts, but a hairline fracture in the scaphoid. Looking at the MRI, he recommended three separate surgical procedures. The first would pin the fracture, the second would drain the cysts and fill each of them with bone grafts, and the third would reposition the displaced tendon.

"What will the estimated recovery period be?" Dr Groopman asked.

"Eighteen to twenty-four months in total," replied Dr B.

Although Dr Groopman was desperate for relief, the idea of undergoing three operations spanning 18 months was not acceptable. He decided to consult a third surgeon, Dr C, one of the most renowned hand surgeons in the US. When Dr Groopman went to see Dr C, he was initially seen by Dr C's assistant. Dr C then came into the room and, while listening to the history from the assistant, examined Dr Groopman's hand. After a couple of minutes, he went to see the X-ray. He came back and said, "We need to do an arthroscopy; I'll have the resident schedule it."

As Dr C turned to leave, Dr Groopman asked, "I wonder if you could tell me what you expect to find with the arthroscopy."

"I'll figure it out when I get in there," he said, and left the room.

Not satisfied with this explanation, Dr Groopman asked the assistant to call Mr C in again. When he returned, Dr Groopman asked him what he thought of a diagnosis.

"Chondrocalcinosis," Dr C replied.

"Wouldn't you see the calcium deposits on the X-rays?" Dr Groopman asked.

"There are cases where the X-rays are negative," Dr C replied.

"And the bone cysts?"

Dr C reiterated that he would figure it out during the procedure, and left the room again.

Dr Groopman was conscious that nothing in any of the tests suggested chondrocalcinosis. He was also aware that even if the diagnosis had been chondrocalcinosis, arthroscopy would not be of any help. Dr C had offered a diagnosis that, while not invented like Dr A's hyper-reactive synovium, was nevertheless unconvincing. Obviously Dr Groopman did not agree to the procedure.

A year later, when he could not bear the pain any longer, Dr Groopman went to a fourth orthopaedic surgeon, Dr D, who surprised Dr Groopman by examining not only his right hand, but also the left one. Dr D X-rayed both hands, not only while the hands were stationary but also when they were in a gripping position. This was the first time anyone had ever paid attention to the left wrist or tried an X-ray of the hands during a manoeuvre. After looking at the X-rays, Dr D concluded that the ligaments between the bones were partially torn and that there were channels within the bone cysts and the joint, which were causing inflammation of the joint. When Dr Groopman mentioned that earlier MRIs had not revealed any of these problems, Dr D replied that, despite the negative MRI findings, he was confident that the ligaments were abnormal and that the connection existed between the cysts and the joints. According to him, surgeons relied too much on such sophisticated investigations; sometimes these had to be discounted if they were out of line with the clinical picture. Dr D then proposed to take bone grafts from the hip, to fill in the cysts and repair the ligament in one operation.

Dr Groopman writes in his book *How Doctors Think* [21] that over the course of three years he consulted many hand surgeons in the US and obtained as many different opinions about what was wrong and what to do, all the time continuing to suffer.

How do you feel after reading this case? Are you not too bothered, perhaps thinking, "It happens – after all, people have different experiences," or are you perturbed by the fact that a Head of the Department of Medicine at Harvard could not get satisfactory treatment for his wrist pain in spite of consulting various surgeons over a period of three years? Let's be clear: the surgeons Dr Groopman consulted were well qualified and competent at their jobs. They had lots of experience and an array of information at their fingertips. Their integrity or ability was not in doubt. But, still, they did not get it right. You cannot dismiss this case by saying that such incidents only happen in the USA. They can happen anywhere, and do. You may already have experienced something like this.

Decision-making lies at the heart of our professional lives. Every day we make decisions – decisions that affect patients' lives. Some are small, others more important. We make mistakes along the way. Indeed, the daunting reality is that important decisions made by intelligent, responsible professionals with the best information and intentions sometimes go wrong. Even good surgeons make bad decisions. Why? How can we reduce the number of bad decisions that are made? More importantly, how can you prevent this problem from affecting you?

The conventional wisdom has been that if you gain more experience, follow evidence-based medicine, implement the protocols, and are analytical in your thinking, then you will make good decisions. Yes, all these methods are of use to a certain extent, but they have their limitations. For example, let's talk about experience. It is a vital issue for surgical trainees due to the changes in the training structure. At the same time, it is just as important for consultants, as, due to the advances in surgical practice, they need to make changes in their practice accordingly.

You may be surprised to hear that experience can be an asset or a liability. As Charles Mayo has said, "...experience can mean doing the wrong thing over and over again." The common argument in favour of experience in decision-making follows this logic: over time, we make mistakes; we learn from those mistakes. We gain experience, and that experience enables us to make better decisions in the future. But what exactly do we mean by experience? Is it age? Is it the length of time spent performing an activity? Or is it an indicator of accumulated expertise? The value of experience in decision-making depends on what you mean by experience. Ideally, experience is repeated feedback that accumulates and becomes developed expertise. Without appropriate feedback, experience would not result in expertise. Therefore, ten years of 'experience' may not reflect ten years of accumulated expertise if you do not improve after the feedback. It may merely be one year of experience repeated ten times! Somebody may have worked in a specialty for some time, but that does not necessarily mean that he/she has had varied experience which has improved to a level of expertise.

We are vulnerable to committing thinking errors. Some thinking errors do not diminish with experience. There are inherent limitations. Firstly, there is a delay in feedback. Because there is typically a long time-lag between making a decision and its outcome, when you take a particular decision during an operation, you might not come to the result within the next few days or weeks or, in some cases, even the next few months. In those cases it is often hard for people to learn from their mistakes. Secondly, people cannot ascertain what the outcome would have been had they made a different choice. You do not perform randomised controlled trials (RCT) for every patient you see, so how can you know how things may have turned out in different circumstances? Learning is not always clear, because we cannot always be sure that what worked in one situation will work in another.

The strongest case for experience lies in its value for assessing situations and for making routine decisions. Experience allows us to size up a situation: "I have seen this situation a number of times before, and I know what has worked, so here is what

I need to do." Experience also works well with routine situations because, again, past practices provide insight into how best to solve a problem. However, experience can reduce the quality of decision-making when it leads to arrogance, overconfidence, or inaccurate perceptions. We see what we expect to see, and extensive experience can limit our perceptions. If our experiences are biased, our perceptions are likely to be inaccurate. Thus, we can fail to perceive problems appropriately.

Expertise can also lead us to view problems in stereotyped ways. The sense of typicality can be so strong that we miss subtle signs of trouble. Or we may know so much that we can explain away those signs. We cannot often see a clear link between cause and effect. Too many variables intervene, and time delays create their own complications. We can learn the wrong lesson from experience. Each time we compile a story about an experience, we run the risk of getting it wrong and stamping in the wrong strategy. In situations where we have fewer opportunities for feedback or the task does not have enough repetitions to build a sense of typicality, we should be cautious about assuming that experience translates into expertise. In these sorts of domains, experience would give us smooth routines, showing that we had been doing the job for a while. Yet our expertise might not go much beyond these surface routines; we would not have a chance to develop reliable expertise.

With all his experience with the orthopaedic surgeons he saw, Dr Groopman went to see Dr Terry Light, who was a former President of the American Society for Surgery of the Hand and also the President of the American Orthopaedic Association. After listening to Dr Groopman's story, Dr Light said, "The key is for everything to add up – the patient's symptoms, the findings on physical examination and what appears meaningful on the MRI or other X-rays. It has to come together and form a coherent picture.....The point is, you have to think of it." Essentially this is another way of saying that it is crucial that a surgeon is able to recognise a pattern. If a surgeon fails to recognise the pattern, he/she gets into trouble. When you are unsure of the pattern, it is wrong to pick up the scalpel and start cutting. Unfortunately this was what surgeons A, B and C were planning to do.

When Dr Groopman asked why it had taken three years for somebody to think of it, Dr Light admitted that he had never really been taught this concept; he learnt instead by observing senior surgeons closely, those who were clear and effective in their judgement and those who were not, and tried then to figure out the key to this difference. He went on to say that although conventional thinking states that surgeons must have great hands, successful surgery is more about skilful decision-making. He acknowledged that there are certain demanding procedures, as in microvascular surgery, that require exquisite dexterity and that most surgeons learn dexterity through repeated practice. "Where they differ most is not in technique, ... but in how they conceptualise a patient's problem and understand what surgery can and cannot do to remedy it. The surgeon's brain is more important than his hands."

Together, Dr Light and Dr Groopman analysed the pitfalls in the thinking of the hand surgeons. Dr A showed a tendency towards action rather than inaction, which is termed 'commission bias' – this occurs when a surgeon is desperate and gives in to the urge to 'do something'. Dr B stopped searching for a diagnosis once he found the bone cysts and the scaphoid fracture on the MRI scan. This is a different cognitive error, called 'search-satisfying error'. Dr C exhibited all the features of overconfident thinking. Dr D avoided this error by continuing to search for answers as he was not satisfied with what was presented in terms of accounting for all the symptoms.

It is not that we are unaware of the uncertainties in surgical practice and have done nothing about it, because we have. We have attempted to address these uncertainties by various means, as mentioned before; we have enriched our knowledge and created an evidence base, among other things. But how far do you think surgical practice is evidence-based? The majority of surgeons would like to answer by saying, "Most of it." However, that would not be an honest reply. Various studies reveal that surgeons do not practice evidence-based medicine (EBM) as much as they would like to believe [22]. Dr. Jack Weinberg has studied surgical decision-making [17]. What he has found is an embarrassing degree of inconsistency in the actions taken by surgeons. His research has shown that the chance of a patient being advised to have a cholecystectomy varied by up to 70%, while recommendations for a hip replacement varied by up to 50%. This reflects the uncertainty in surgical practice, with the varied experience and attitudes of individual surgeons leading to massively different surgical management. Although the knowledge of what the right thing to do often exists, we still frequently fail to do it. Informed knowledge has simply not made its way far enough into actual practice. Overall, compliance with various evidence-based guidelines ranges from over 70% of patients to less than 20% in others. The grey areas in surgery are considerable. Every day we confront situations in which clear evidence of what to do is missing, and yet choices must be made. Exactly which patients with back pain should be treated by surgery and which by conservative measures? For many cases, the answers can be obvious, but for many others, we simply do not know. In the absence of evidence about what to do for a particular patient, you learn in surgery to make decisions based on your personal experience.

In virtually all arenas of surgical practice, the data to guide decisions are ill-defined and the use and extent of care is driven by surgeons' individual preferences and choices. A study entitled 'Analysis of the decision-making process leading to appendectomy' evaluated this variability [23]. Decisions on appendicectomy are among the most common in the surgical field. However, the frequency seems to differ considerably between hospitals and counties. In Sweden, the average appendicectomy frequency is 1.27 per thousand people, with a variation between different areas ranging from 0.6 to 1.9 [24]. In hospitals in the county of Varmland, differences in appendicectomy frequency of between 0.64 and 1.40 per thousand people were noted. No significant socio-demographic differences exist between the regions with the highest and lowest frequencies. This raises the question of whether the differences reflect different surgical decision-making cultures. This is a strong example of a lack of evidence-based practice at ground level.

One day, I was waiting in the surgeon's room of an operating theatre when I overheard a conversation between three surgeons. I gathered that they were discussing a complication experienced by their colleague: a leak following an emergency sigmoid resection and primary anastomosis for sigmoid diverticulitis with contained contamination.

"Clearly," said Mr Wilson, "this was a serious lapse of judgement. I cannot imagine what he was thinking when he decided to put the colon back together again. He put his patient at risk unnecessarily."

"I do not agree," said Mr Lewis. "There is good evidence that anastomoses can be performed safely on an unprepared bowel. This was a recognised complication, and simply reflects the fact that we will never eliminate complications entirely."

"Maybe," said Mr Smith, "but data from experimental studies shows that faecal loading impairs anastomotic healing. The approach may be safe in ideal circumstances, but not in a man who has known comorbidities. I would not have attempted an anastomosis here."

"The point is," said Mr Wilson, "that, in the real world, patients are not experimental rats or carefully chosen subjects who are enrolled in clinical trials, but are living, breathing humans who have plenty of associated health problems, who are operated on not by ultra specialists in tertiary centres, but by surgeons like you and me. You do not take chances; you do the safest thing possible, and, for me, that would have been a Hartmann's procedure."

While I waited in the coffee room I started to wonder – did the surgeon err in his judgement? What would have been the safest course of action? What would have been best for the patient? Is there a right answer, and how can we ever know?

Why is it so difficult to practise evidence-based surgery? The reasons are associated with the nature of surgical practice as well as the nature of surgeons themselves. For ardent EBM critics, the literature is flawed due to non-pragmatic studies, editorial bias and lack of generalisability. They find it hard to accept that we depend on a body of knowledge that is so heavily criticised. The issue for others is the question of what acceptable evidence would be in a surgical context, since there are some aspects of surgery that are suitable for an RCT, but there are also some that are not. The critics also object to the concept of EBM, as, according to them, it devalues their clinical experience.

It was thought that surgeons were not compliant because of their lack of knowledge about EBM. However, it was realised that the problem cannot be attributed entirely to ignorance. Telling people about evidence-based medicine is an ineffective method of changing practice. Didactic 'talk and chalk' sessions in lecture halls or a 'bums on seats' approach in tutorial rooms does not change surgeons' behaviour [25]. Information may be necessary for professional behavioural change, but it is rarely, if ever, sufficient. So, the question remains: how do we influence surgeons' behaviour to promote evidence-based practice? Marteau has studied this problem; he says that we have to make use of psychological strategies to bring about effective change. And, for that to happen, we need to understand how surgeons think in clinical situations.

Why are some surgeons slow to adopt evidence-based practice? The answer is down to the way those surgeons think. The style of surgeons' thinking creates either barriers or an easy path to the implementation of evidence-based practice. For example, some personality traits are associated with the inclination to try out and use innovations. Some people are more set in their ways than others. Some individuals will need more input and will take more time to change [26]. Implementation of best practice for a patient in front of you is a complex phenomenon and we need to have a better understanding of how surgeons think in the clinical context. We consider surgery as a scientific discipline and we are supposed to use scientific thinking to treat our patients. However, when you are managing a patient in front of you, it is not just analytical thinking that you use. The realities of clinical life are much more than just a science. Even as a science, surgery is changing rapidly. The information generated is enormous and difficult to keep pace with. To make the decision on the ground we have to act on incomplete and uncertain information. There is a gap between the available information and your aim. Because of this gap between our resources and our aims, surgeons need to be aware of the limitations of surgery as a science and the limitations of their own thinking. The clinical information may be insufficient; at the same time, one's knowledge cannot be assumed to be up to date. There is a problem of applying the knowledge in addition to not having sufficient knowledge. In many situations, surgeons are aware of what should be done and also the best way in which it could be done, yet they do not always succeed in application. The number of errors that occur in hospitals indicates that knowledge was available but was not applied due to difficulties in decision-making. Why?

We often hear that we live in the information age, and this new age can come with information overload. Quantity of information, however, is not synonymous with quality. In making complex decisions, we often seek out more information, because we associate more with better. The continual search for more information can result in needless delays or even complete inertia. When you are fearful of making a decision, it's easy to rationalise postponement by arguing that you need more information to make an intelligent decision. The effective decision maker learns to know when enough is enough. He is also able to differentiate quality from quantity. The effective decision maker accepts that he is almost never going to have all the information he wants in order to make a decision. Uncertainty is part of life and part of decision-making. You can't eliminate uncertainty. You just want to acquire an appropriate amount of information to minimise it.

The cerebral flaw has been exacerbated by modernity. We live in a culture that is awash with information; this is the age of Google, PDAs and online encyclopaedias. We get anxious whenever we are cut off from all this knowledge, as if it is impossible for anyone to make a decision without a search engine. But this abundance comes with some hidden costs. The main problem is that the human brain was not designed to deal with such a flood of data. As a result, we are constantly exceeding the capacity of our prefrontal cortices. Some studies have shown that, of two groups, the group that had less information performed better than the group that had far more information. It proves the saying that "a wealth of information creates a poverty of attention." Sometimes, knowledge has diminishing returns; right up until it has negative returns. This is a counter-intuitive idea. When making decisions, people almost always assume that more information is better. But it is important to know the limitations of this approach, which are rooted in the limitations of the brain. The brain can only handle so much information at any one time, so when a person gives the brain too many facts and then asks it to make a decision based on the facts that seem important, the person in question is asking for trouble.

I remember a story I was told while I was working in the USA.

A surgeon noticed that his orders were not being followed by a particular nurse. One day the surgeon called the nurse into his cabin. As she stepped in, the surgeon asked her to go out and read what was on his cabin door. The nurse, perplexed by the surgeon's behaviour, told the surgeon that she saw his name on the door.

"No, you have missed the most important thing written there."

Now, more embarrassed than perplexed, the nurse left the room again and, upon returning, said that she saw his qualifications, 'MD'.

"Yes," said the surgeon, "that's the most important thing. Do you know what 'MD' stands for? It stands for 'Make Decision'. The 'MD' reminds people like you that I am a surgeon and that I am the one who makes decisions – you just follow them."

(You would have thought that the saga would end there. But it did not. The following day, the nurse went to the surgeon and said, "Do you know what the RN on my badge stands for? It stands for 'Reject Nonsense'.")

Sure, the surgeon knew very well that making decisions is a hallmark of being a surgeon. But he did not know how to put this into practice sensibly: he had not learnt how to execute the decisions. In fact, none of us are formally taught how to make decisions or how to improve our decision-making skills. There are very few things in our professional lives that are as important as the quality of our decisions. From clinical outcomes to your overall job satisfaction, the results are largely due to the decisions you make. However, we are not aware that decision-making is a skill that needs to be honed, just like any other technical skill. In spite of the importance of making good decisions, you do not receive explicit training in decision-making. We assume that, with clinical practice and experience, we can learn to be good decision makers. But, as we have seen earlier, experience is not necessarily very helpful in this case. Studies reveal that many people do not make good decisions, even after gaining experience. It is interesting to note that as a surgeon you cannot qualify without the knowledge of basic sciences like anatomy or physiology. However, you can skip the basic understanding of decision science, which you need to apply to every patient. Do you know why some surgeons make better decisions than others, or how decision-making skills affect surgical outcomes? Surgery as a specialty and surgeons as individuals have not taken decision-making seriously enough – not as seriously as the aviation industry and pilots have.

The aviation industry did not take decision-making or human factors seriously until the 1980s. Despite a long list of aviation reforms, the percentage of pilot errors refused to budge from 1940 to 1990, holding steady at around 70%. It didn't matter what type of plane was being flown or where the plane was going. The fact remained: most aviation deaths were due to bad decisions by the pilots. From the early 1990s, the percentage of crashes attributed to pilot error began to decline rapidly. According to the most current statistics, mistakes by pilots are responsible for less than 30% of all plane accidents, with a 70% reduction in the number of accidents caused by poor decision-making. The result is that flying has become safer than ever. The most dangerous part of travelling on a commercial aeroplane is the drive to the airport.

What caused this dramatic reduction in pilot error? One of the crucial factors in the dramatic decline in pilot error was the development of a decision-making strategy known as crew resource management (CRM). In recent years, CRM has moved beyond the cockpit. Many hospitals have realised that the same decision-making techniques that can prevent pilot error can also prevent mistakes during surgery.

The safety of flights is a testament to the possibility of improvement. The reduction in the pilot-error rate is a powerful reminder that mistakes are not inevitable, and that planes do not have to crash. As the modern cockpit demonstrates, a few simple innovations and a little self-awareness can dramatically improve the way people think, so that the brain system is used in its ideal context. The aviation industry took decision-making seriously – making a science of pilot error – and the result has been a stunning advance in performance.

The first step towards making better decisions is to see ourselves as we really are: to look inside the black box of the human brain. We need to honestly assess our flaws and talents, our strengths and shortcomings. For the first time, such vision is possible. We finally have tools that can pierce the mystery of the mind, revealing the intricate machinery that shapes our behaviour. Now we need to put this knowledge to work.

Key points

- Experience is necessary to acquire surgical expertise; however, obtaining experience does not automatically or necessarily make you an expert.

- Although we would like to believe it, the practice of evidence-based medicine has not percolated to a satisfactory level.

- The first step in improving decision-making is to understand what it is.

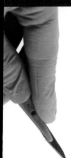

Chapter 4

Cognitive errors –
what were you thinking then?

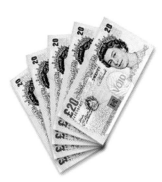

Problems in thought processes, including mistakes in decision-making, are the major factors contributing to surgical errors. Understanding these biases and errors would be an initial step for anyone who intends to improve their decision-making skills. This is important for two reasons. First, the biases offer clues to the thinking process underlying decision-making, and, secondly, they indicate areas where improvement is needed.

Imagine a situation in which you have received £100.

If you were asked to choose only one option from the following two choices, which one would you choose?

A – You receive an additional £50.

Or

B – A coin is tossed:

If it is heads, you receive an additional £100.

If it is tails, you receive nothing more.

Please choose your answer – A or B.

Now imagine that you have received £200.

If you were asked to choose only one option from the following two choices, which one would you choose?

C – You must pay back £50 immediately.

Or

D – A coin is tossed:

If it is heads, you pay back nothing.

If it is tails, you pay back £100.

Please choose your answer – C or D.

What were your choices? If you are like others, you might have chosen A and D. That is how the majority of people respond when asked to take part in this exercise.

If you look more closely, you may realise that all four choices - A, B, C and D - are of equal value [27]. This can be explained as follows:

In the first scenario, the two choices are: a 100% chance that you would have 50% extra money, i.e. Choice A = 150 (100 + 50); or a 50% chance that you would have 100% extra money, i.e. Choice B = 150 (100 + 50 [100% .5 = 50]); to ascertain the value of a choice the total value is divided by the total number of options.

In the second scenario, again, there are two choices: a 100% chance that you will lose £50, i.e. Choice C = 150 (200 - 50); or a 50% chance that you will lose £100, i.e. Choice D = 150 (200 - 50 [100% .5 = 50]).

Since all choices have the value of 150, you would imagine that, if this scenario was presented to a number of people, their responses would be distributed evenly between all four choices. For example, out of 100 responses, each choice would be selected approximately 25 (+/- 5) times. It doesn't happen that way. Interestingly, it is seen that the majority of people have a strong preference for A and D. Cognitive researchers do not observe an equal distribution: they observe peaks at A and D. Why do people make different choices in spite of being given similar value options?

These choices symbolise two types of behaviour: one is 'risk-taking' behaviour and the other is 'risk-avoiding' behaviour. Choices A and C indicate risk-avoiding, while choices B and D indicate risk-taking behaviour. Some individuals are risk-takers, and choose B and D, while some are risk averse, choosing options A and C. That is straightforward. What is not straightforward is that the majority of people choose option A in the first scenario – in other words, avoid risk – but become risk-takers in the second case and choose option D.

What is the difference between the two scenarios? In the first scenario, the person would be gaining money, while in the second scenario he/she would be losing money. So the difference is in the context of gain or loss. In a situation where there is a gain, people tend to avoid risk. That is why the majority of people opt for choice A in the first scenario. They want to avoid the risk of not getting additional money. However, in a situation where there is a loss, people are willing to take a risk, and therefore the majority of people choose D in the second case.

This exercise reveals our thinking process when making decisions. We think that we make decisions by thinking rationally. The value of these four choices is equal only if you use pure rational thinking. However, the values change and become unequal when psychological factors creep into these choices. We are not conscious of the influence of psychological factors. Although we consider ourselves rational thinkers, in life, it is not just logic that we use when taking decisions. Like it or not, emotions creeps into our thinking and affect our decisions.

Is it just ordinary, lay people who change their decisions because of emotional factors? If you think that well-educated professionals like doctors would not succumb to these soft approaches, take a look at the next scenario.

Case scenario 1

You are in charge of a medical unit that is preparing for an outbreak of a new strain of swine flu, which is expected to kill 600 people in your region. Two plans to combat the outbreak are available to you. If you choose plan A, 200 people will definitely be saved. If you choose plan B, there is a 1/3 probability that all 600 people will be saved. Which plan would you choose? Plan A or Plan B?

Case scenario 2

You are in charge of a medical unit that is preparing for an outbreak of a new strain of swine flu, which is expected to kill 600 people in your region. Two plans to combat the outbreak are available. If you choose plan C, 400 people will definitely die. If you choose plan D, there is a 2/3 probability that all 600 people will die. Which plan would you choose? Plan C or Plan D?

Have you noted that in both scenarios the number of people saved is 200, irrespective of whether plan A, B, C or D is chosen? Since there is no difference between these outcomes, there should not be a major preference among the choices. Doctors, nonetheless, respond differently to the two scenarios. In the first scenario more doctors choose A, while in the second scenario they choose D. You may have noticed that although the outcomes are the same, they are presented in two different frames. The first one is the 'lives saved' frame and the second is the 'lives lost' frame. Thus, the first is a 'gain' scenario and the second is a 'loss' scenario. Similar to the previous example, doctors' choices vary according to the 'saved' or the 'died' frame. In the 'lives saved' frame, they prefer plan A, i.e. definitely save 200 people, while in the 'lives lost' frame they prefer choice D, the more risky choice of there being a 2/3 probability that all 600 people will die. Thus, in a clinical situation, if there is a potential gain (lives saved), doctors do not take risks, but in a situation of potential loss, they prefer to take risks [28].

The two scenarios depicted above differ only in the manner in which words are used. Nevertheless, just a change in the wording affects the choice in the scenario. The way in which choices are described influences the decision more than you would imagine. We can see this happening in our clinical practice. Even a subtle difference in presentation has a significant impact. Suppose you have a cancer patient who has to take a decision about his treatment. His decision will be different if you tell him "There is a 30% chance of you dying within a year of the surgery" as compared to, "There is a 70% chance of you living more than a year after the surgery."

It is not just patients whose decisions are affected by frames. Doctors are also influenced by the framing effect when making clinical decisions. In a research experiment [29], doctors were asked to choose between surgical and radiation treatment for a cancer patient. In one scenario, the clinical outcome was described in terms of survival rates. The other scenario described the same outcome, but as mortality rates. In other words, 'surgery has a 30% survival rate' was a typical example for the survival frame and 'surgery has a 70% mortality rate' as an example for the mortality frame. The treatments described two outcomes: immediate and five years. Radiation was shown to have a higher immediate survival rate, but a lower five-year survival rate compared to surgery. Although the survival and mortality rates described the same information, the doctors expressed different preferences in relation to the two frames. In the survival frame, they preferred surgery, while in the mortality frame they preferred radiation. The higher immediate mortality from the surgery had a larger impact on choice in the mortality frame, thus reducing its preference. This just highlights the fact that, even when making clinical decisions, the manner in which the description is framed affects our decisions in some cases. Cognitive scientists call this a 'framing bias'.

In a paper entitled 'Do clinicians always maximise patient outcomes? A conjoint analysis of references for carotid artery testing' [30], Frankel Sassi showed that the value clinicians place on diagnostic information is subject to psychological influence and framing biases, which affect patient outcomes. They assessed the relative value attached by surgeons to different diagnostic test characteristics and how their preferences related to patient outcomes. Results showed that the preference was for positive predictive value (PPV), relative to negative predictive value (NPV). They concluded that surgeons attach substantially more importance to positive predictive value of carotid artery tests than would be justified by their impact on patient outcomes. Cognitive errors and attitudes to risk play an important role in explaining this finding.

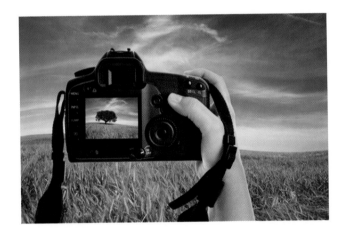

The term 'framing' is better appreciated from a photographic point of view. When the photographer aims the camera at the object, he views the object through the frame. He wants to put the object at the centre of the frame. He focuses the lens – and, by that, his attention – on what he believes is the most relevant point. Framing is a technique we use to see and understand the situation, be it by vision or by words. The words we use shape the frames through which we perceive the situation. By choosing certain words, we change the way in which we see a given situation. When you want to make a decision, you do the same thing when you define the problem and review your options. The way you define or perceive the problems affects the solution. Frames determine which aspect of the situation will be attended to and which will be filtered out.

Here is an interesting story of how a decision was changed by taking advantage of framing bias. Two young priests were heavy smokers and somewhat troubled about this habit when they were praying.

The first asked his bishop, "Would it be permissible for me to smoke while praying to the Lord?"

"No," said the bishop.

After a few days, the second priest asked the bishop the same question, but worded it differently. "During the moments of weakness when I smoke, would it be permissible for me to say a prayer to the Lord?"

"Yes, of course, my son," said the priest.

Next time you are on the ward, compare the differences in management between two terminally-ill patients, one of whom has been declared as DNR (do not resuscitate). It has been observed that DNR patients receive less-than-optimum treatment for symptoms like pain, insomnia, and infection – purely because the frame has been changed from 'for resuscitation' to 'not for resuscitation'.

Bias, in general, is a tendency towards a particular view. In social life we see cultural bias, racial bias, or regional bias. In the scientific domain we come across sampling bias, observer's bias, publication bias, and so on. Fundamentally, biased thinking is deep-rooted in our thinking – so deeply rooted that it takes effort to bring it to the surface. We think that, with our knowledge and intelligence, we are able to avoid such bias. Anybody who has sufficient experience in clinical practice will agree that this is not the case. The next example supports this statement.

Case scenario

A 40-year-old male patient, who was working as a fitness instructor in a gymnasium, came to the emergency department with complaints of chest pain a few hours before. He was seen by the A&E registrar. The patient's assessment did not reveal any other symptoms apart from retrosternal chest pain. The registrar went over the checklist of risk factors for cardiac diseases, but did not find any. Being a fitness instructor, the patient was leading a very healthy lifestyle and was in excellent physical health. The clinical examination, cardiogram and other investigations, including cardiac enzymes, came back as normal. The patient was reassured that the pain must be of muscular origin and that it was OK for him to go home. Eight hours after he was sent home from A&E, he was readmitted to the hospital with a massive myocardial infarction.

Did the registrar miss the diagnosis? If he did, was it due to lack of knowledge or negligence? Actually, it was neither. When this case was discussed later, it became apparent that the registrar was a victim of what is called 'representative bias'. He put his blind faith in his (wrong) thinking. His thinking at the time of diagnosis was over-influenced by looking at the patient's healthy lifestyle and very fit body. If he had ignored his biased thinking, he may have realised that the patient could have an unstable angina and the laboratory investigations in the window period may be reported as normal. Since the patient's presentation did not match with the 'risky' category, the registrar concluded that he did not need further monitoring. In cases of representative bias, like this one, thinking is guided by prototypes, so possibilities that contradict the prototype are not considered.

One of the heuristics most surgeons are aware of is: "If it looks like a duck, walks like a duck, and quacks like a duck, it's a duck." Our pattern recognition is related to this maxim, which is called 'representativeness'. In pattern recognition, you match the patient's signs and symptoms with the template in your mind and look for matching or representativeness. After matching the patient's characteristics, we put the patient into the diagnostic category. Like other heuristics, this strategy works most of the time. It allows us to organise information in the appropriate manner so that we can recognise the pattern. However, if we rely blindly on this strategy, there is a risk of overseeing atypical presentation. You may miss a diagnosis in a particular case if you (wrongly) feel that the patient does not represent a particular class.

Representativeness bias illustrates the way we reason. When confronted with a decision, we tend to look for aspects of the decision that are similar to previous decisions we have made. We then use the simplifying analogy that worked for past decisions. However, the analogy or the apparent similarity we use may not be appropriate for the current situation. You may have read the warning at the bottom of the investment brochure: "Past performance of the fund cannot guarantee future performance."

Our memory, formed by past experience, has some similarities to the current situation, but it may have some differences also. We can be misled into forming a view of the situation that is misguided. This misguided view leads us to take the wrong course of action. When we have been very successful in the past, we often presume that our actions will again be successful. In such situations we find it hard to question ourselves and correct our errors. In some cases, when people are challenged about their (wrong) thoughts, they produce an apparently plausible explanation for the inappropriate decision. It may not be an explanation that will convince an objective listener, but it is enough to convince the person giving the explanation. In other words, the person whose decision is influenced by biased thinking will not believe that it is.

Heuristics

Inappropriate decisions are made because of deviations in the thinking process. Biases sneak into our decision-making processes. They come out of our attempts to find shortcuts. Most of us are busy in our day-to-day clinical work; our lives are complicated and we can't spend all our time thinking and analysing everything. When we have to make judgements, we use simple rules of thumb to help us to make a decision. We use rules of thumb because, most of the time, they are quick and useful. In many cases, these shortcuts are helpful. However, they can also lead to severe distortions of the thinking process. Some people learn the tricks to manage the thinking process. They know their biases and have figured out how to minimise their impact. The scientific term for a rule of thumb is a 'heuristic'. Heuristics are short statements that guide our thinking. You can say that heuristics are short statements drawn on long experiences! Some heuristics are handed over to us by other experienced surgeons and some we develop from our own experience. Heuristics are methods of solving problems when no formula exists. Such tricks of the trade are informal and are based on experience. They are informal because iteration, such as the repeated performance of an operation, results in the unconscious development of techniques for overcoming problems. Heuristics are important contributors to experience and, to the uninitiated, they may appear to be trivial, for example, the use of packs to provide exposure, the use of tissue tension to facilitate dissection, and the way that fingers are used to expose a bleeding vessel [31]. All experienced surgeons have such traits and they collectively contribute to a style of operating. Risk management cannot advance without a genuine understanding of how surgeons work, and this requires a greater appreciation of heuristics. The mental heuristics that experienced surgeons use to minimise risk are usually expressed in the form of anecdotes. This is why informal talk between operations and in the lifts and corridors during rounds are so important; they help to socialise trainees into the profession of surgery.

Availability heuristics

Earlier we saw how we use representativeness heuristics to access our memories for reasoning; there is another heuristic we use to access our memories, which is known as the availability heuristic. You may be aware of the heuristics "the sound of hoof beats means horses ... (and not zebras)" and "common things are common". We use these rules of thumb in practice, either consciously or unconsciously, and they can work – not always, though. When we use such heuristics inappropriately, we overestimate a probability. Here is an example. You see a patient complaining of abdominal pain. You struggle to find out the cause of his abdominal pain. After various investigations, it turns out that the patient has porphyria. You are excited to have come across a rare cause of abdominal pain. After a few days you see another patient with abdominal pain. The memories of your previous patient come to mind, and one of the early diagnoses you consider is porphyria. You think of porphyria as a possible diagnosis even though you may be aware that porphyria is a very rare entity.

Here is another case.

Case scenario

A 65-year-old male patient went to see his GP, complaining of breathing difficulties. Over the preceding few weeks, many patients from the surgery had gone to the hospital with viral pneumonia. The GP noted that the patient had a low-grade fever and his respiratory rate was 30/min. Auscultation did not provide any further information. The GP sent the patient to the hospital with a diagnosis of viral pneumonia. In the hospital he was seen by the SHO, John, who confirmed the GP's findings and ordered further investigations. The investigations showed a normal WBC count, but the electrolytes showed an acid-base imbalance with a shift towards acid. His chest X-ray did not show characteristic white streaks of viral pneumonia. John had admitted quite a few cases of viral pneumonia over the preceding days. He made a diagnosis of sub-clinical viral pneumonia and admitted this patient. Before he finished his duty, John handed the patient over to the on-call SHO. During the handover, when the colleague asked about the patient's diagnosis, John explained that although the patient's investigations were negative for pneumonia, for him the diagnosis was clear. The investigations were negative as the presentation was sub-clinical. The following day, when John returned to the ward, he saw that overnight the patient's diagnosis had changed from sub-clinical pneumonia to 'aspirin toxicity'. Surprised by the diagnosis, John explored the events during his absence. He found out that the on-call SHO had reviewed the case in the evening. It became apparent that the patient, thinking he was suffering from a cold, had taken a few aspirin. John had not bothered to ask what he meant by "a few" – the fact was that the patient had taken a few dozen aspirin tablets that day. The presentation – rapid breathing and the shift in electrolytes – was due to aspirin toxicity and not viral sub-clinical pneumonia.

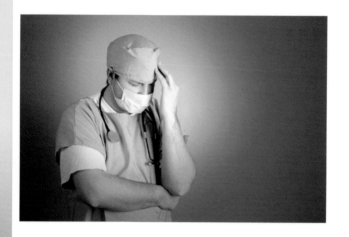

This case reveals how John committed various cognitive errors. One of them was 'availability bias'. Availability, in this context, is the tendency to consider a diagnosis just because it comes to mind easily. For John, the diagnosis of sub-clinical pneumonia was readily available because he had seen many cases of pneumonia over the preceding weeks. This easy availability of a diagnostic entity was one of the factors that led to the incorrect diagnosis.

A hospital prepared a software program to reduce the costs of investigations. When doctors were about to order an expensive investigation, the cost of that investigation used to flash up on the computer screen. Just the cost price – nothing else! Interestingly, this flash resulted in doctors ordering the test less often and saved the hospital money. Not that the doctors didn't know the cost of the investigation before it flashed in front of them – they did. But it didn't affect their decisions, as it was not available to them when making the decision. However, when the information was available to the brain at the time of the decision, that availability had an impact on the decision.

We tend to remember the events that are most available in our memory – those that are most recent and vivid. This, in turn, distorts our ability to consider events in a balanced manner [32]. One example of this phenomenon relates to the fear of flying. The evidence shows that flying on a commercial airline is one of the safest forms of transport. You are far more likely to die in a car than in a plane. The probability of dying in a plane is one in 11 million compared to one in 5,000 for dying in a car crash, yet millions of people don't believe these numbers. Why? Because when a plane goes down and people die, it makes headlines. The stories and pictures of these accidents grab at our emotions and become indelibly marked in our memories. The media coverage given to dramatic events tends to make them more available in our memories, and as a result we tend to think they are more frequent than they are.

The quality of the information available at the time of the decision has an additional impact. Surgical cognition has a significant component of visual thinking. In the case of visual thinking, the more vivid the image is, the more impact it will have on our thinking. Suppose you have seen a routine case, but the image of that case is still vivid in your mind – that vividness would add to your thinking process on a subconscious level.

In a paper analysing medical decision-making, Dr Potchen concluded that what most influenced clinical decisions was "the last bad experience" [33]. He conducted a study regarding mammographies and breast biopsies. A certain percentage of patients undergoing a mammography undergo a further biopsy. In theory, not more than 5% of women undergoing a mammography should need further biopsies. In practice, however, the acceptable norm would be up to 10%. What Dr Potchen found was that some radiologists referred up to 15% of cases for biopsy – 50% above the average. What he discovered was that the radiologists who referred more than an average number of patients had been sued for not picking up on malignant cases and thus had had "a bad experience". The consequence of missing a malignant lesion and being sued had affected the radiologists' thinking. The emotional factor attached to this issue made this information more available at the time of a decision. Similar to the software that would flash-up the cost of the investigation on the computer screen, memories of the bad experience used to flash up in these radiologists' minds and change their behaviour.

Heuristics of unpacking

Here is an example of a different type of availability heuristic called unpacking.

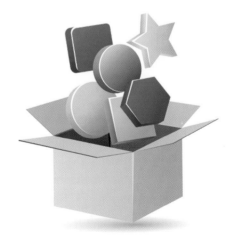

Case scenario A

You have seen a 22-year-old woman with a right lower-quadrant abdominal pain of 12 hours' duration.

Estimate the probability of the following diagnoses:

1) Gastroenteritis   --------%
2) Ectopic pregnancy   --------%
3) None of the above   --------%

                           Total   100 %

Case scenario B

You have seen a 22-year-old woman with a right lower-quadrant abdominal pain of 12 hours' duration.

Estimate the probability of the following diagnoses:

1) Gastroenteritis   --------%
2) Ectopic pregnancy   --------%
3) Appendicitis   --------%
4) Pyelonephritis   --------%
5) Pelvic inflammatory disease   --------%
6) None of the above   --------%

                         Total   100 %

We gave the two scenarios above to two groups of surgeons. As you can see, the second set has three additional options. It is reasonable to expect that the additional three options in the second set should be considered while you are tackling the first scenario. Thus, you would include them in the 'none of the above' list, making the percentage of the 'none of the above' category bigger in the first scenario than in the second one [34]. To make it simpler, I would say that 'none of the above' in the first scenario should include the percentage of the number of appendicitis, pyelonephritis and pelvic inflammatory disease cases, as those diagnoses should be considered in that scenario. However, we observed that surgeons considered those diagnoses only when they were mentioned in the second scenario.

We think a particular diagnosis is more likely if it is described explicitly and thus is made available to our minds. The more specific a description we receive, the more strongly we think of the diagnosis. If all the various possibilities in a problem space are not specified (are not unpacked), we have a tendency to ignore them. Unpacking is a strategy to improve the availability of all possibilities and events. This principle can be observed while we are making a request for a radiological investigation. If we are sending a patient for a CT scan of the head, and among the provisional diagnoses we just write 'neoplasm', the radiologist's thinking may not spread widely enough. On the other hand, if we write other possibilities that we are considering, such as intra-cerebral or subarachnoid haemorrhage or cavernous sinus thrombosis, he may be able to consider other options. When more possibilities are raised, the probability of finding something increases.

One important corollary to this availability heuristic is in regard to visual thinking. When people are asked to imagine an outcome, they tend to think of it as more likely than people who were not asked to imagine the specific outcome. If group A were asked to visualise a specific event and then asked how likely that event is to occur, and group B were asked whether the same specific outcome were likely without being asked to visualise it first, then the members of group A tend to view the event as more likely than group B.

One of the types of judgements surgeons make is to estimate the probability of an event. For example, how appropriate would the chosen surgical approach be? How likely is it that the thyroid would have a retrosternal extension? When asked to predict an event, one imagines that event, watches its outcome and then makes a prediction. It has been observed that the more vividly we can imagine the connection between cause and effect, the more probable the event appears to be for us. Thus, the prediction depends on an imagined connection between cause and effect, which may not in fact be true. For example, in an experiment [35] in which people were asked to think of the probability that the next earthquake would cause a flood in their city, they came up with an estimate of a 30% chance that the earthquake would cause a flood. Later they were asked to consider the probability that the next earthquake would cause a dam to break and flood the area; they said that there was a 100% chance that the earthquake would cause a flood. Thus, the second probability was higher than the first, which is illogical, because the second event (an earthquake breaks the dam and causes a flood) is actually included in the first scenario (an earthquake causes a flood). Moreover, because an earthquake can cause a flood without breaking a dam, the more general statement has in fact a higher probability of causing floods. Logically, the probability estimation for the first event should be higher than for the second event. The explanation for why people increased the probability in the second scenario is that people found visualising that situation easier than visualising the first one. The more detailed the description of the event is, the more likely people are to imagine it easily and specifically.

Essentially, the availability heuristic operates on the notion that, if you can think of it, it must be important. We judge the frequency, probability or likely cause of an event by the degree to which instances of that event are readily available in the memory, rather than by careful assessment of all the data. A memory may be available because it evokes an emotion, is vivid, is easily imagined, or is specific. Vivid, emotional, or easily imagined events are more likely to be brought into focus by our brain than equally relevant events that have neutral emotions. Personal experiences are going to be more vivid and more specific than stories we have been told or material we have been taught. The availability heuristic has other associated sub-effects. The recency bias claims that we access recent information more than older information, even if the older information is more relevant. Experience is not in itself a problem. Decision makers who recognise they are doing something unfamiliar will normally be cautious and put in place an appropriate decision process. They will seek experts, involve others and increase the amount of analysis. The problem with a lack of relevant experience is that it opens the door to misleading experiences.

At this point, it is important to clarify that the basic thinking process for heuristics and bias is the same. The difference between them is about appropriate application. Both mechanisms work at a subconscious level. They could be considered as software used for a particular application. It works automatically. What we see is the result. The term 'bias' in this context is not the term 'bias' that we use in day-to-day life. When we say that somebody is biased, we assume that the person is conscious of the bias. The biases, from a cognitive science point of view, are not conscious. It also needs to be clarified that bias is not the same as self-interest. Suppose you are consciously avoiding taking a particular decision because you are worried about the consequences. That is not biased thinking. If you take a decision without being overtly conscious, it would be biased thinking. The point needs to be highlighted that it is unlikely that you are aware of your biased thinking unless you specifically explore it.

Confirmation bias

In addition to availability bias, John, the SHO who diagnosed sub-clinical viral pneumonia, also committed what is called confirmation bias. Instead of integrating all the key information, he picked only a few features of the patient's illness: his fever, increased respiratory rate, and the shift in acid-base balance. He rationalised the contradictory data – the absence of any extra findings, normal white blood counts – as simply being due to the earlier stage of pneumonia. In fact, these discrepancies should have signalled to him that his thinking was wrong. Such cherry-picking of the information is termed 'confirmation bias'.

We assume that we gather information objectively. But we don't. We gather information selectively. We seek out information that reaffirms our choices, and we discount information that contradicts judgements. We also tend to accept information at face value that confirms our preconceived views, while being critical and sceptical of information that challenges these views. This confirmation bias influences where we go to collect evidence, because we tend to seek out places that are more likely to tell us what we want to hear. It also leads us to give too much weight to supporting evidence and too little to contradictory information.

This type of thinking can also be described as 'I hear what I want to hear' thinking. This bias is seen as a tendency to look for confirming evidence to support your diagnosis, rather than looking for disconfirming evidence to refute it. In some situations, we choose to neglect disconfirming evidence, because, if we accept it, we may have to start our thinking process all over again. As a sheer avoidance of going through that process, we focus on the data that confirms our diagnosis. This bias may seriously compound errors that may arise from anchoring (discussed later), where a prematurely concluded diagnosis is inappropriately strengthened. It also leads to the perseverance of diagnoses that were weak in the first place, and may lead to the correct diagnosis, and thus appropriate treatment, being missed. When situations are ambiguous, what you perceive depends upon your perception more than the situation itself. Your attitudes and interests affect what you see. The clinical circumstances can be far more ambiguous than most of us are willing to admit, and each of us has a unique perceptual base from which we see and interpret these situations. The result is that we are incapable of objectively seeing events around us. Rather, what we do is selectively interpret events based on our biased perceptions, and then call this interpretation reality. Selective perception biases decision-making by influencing the information we pay attention to, the problems we identify, and the alternatives we develop.

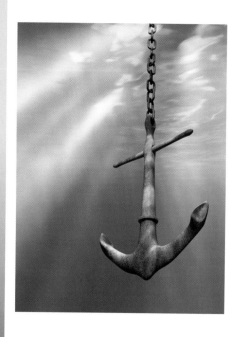

Anchoring bias

When John, the medical SHO in the sub-clinical viral pneumonia case, asked the patient whether he had taken any medication, the patient replied, "A few aspirin." John did not bother to ask what a few meant; he took this information as further evidence for his diagnosis that the patient had a viral syndrome which began as a cold and had then developed into pneumonia. Another thinking error John made was 'anchoring'.

Anchoring is a short-cut in thinking, when you jump to a single conclusion without considering other possibilities. This is like a sailor throwing down the anchor of the ship, with the confidence that he has thrown it down just where it needs to be. When he looks at the map to check, his confirmation bias allows him to see only the landmark he expects or wants to see and means that he ignores those that should tell him that in fact the ship is still at sea. You selectively survey the data, driven by the expectation that your initial diagnosis is correct. This strengthens your conviction.

The anchoring effect is actually a common consumer phenomenon. Consider the price tags in a car showroom. Nobody actually pays the prices listed in the bold black ink on the windows. The inflated sticker is merely an anchor that allows the car salesperson to make the real price of the car seem like a better deal. When a person is offered the inevitable discount, the person is convinced that the car is a bargain. In essence, the anchoring effect is about the brain's spectacular inability to dismiss irrelevant information.

The anchoring effect is most potent when there is a lack of objective information to compare against. In ambiguous situations, we need to be particularly cautious of trivial factors, because they can have a profound effect on anchoring us to an initial position that is hard to deviate from.

Anchoring relates to the fact that, rather than confronting the operator out of the blue, accidents evolve. Hence, the proficient expert surgeon makes initial decisions with the full realisation that these may change if, or as, the situation evolves, and thus is able to revise his or her strategy as dictated by the situation through an updating feedback process. Anchoring occurs when this revision process fails and the surgeon remains fixed on an erroneous assessment of the situation, unable to revise the strategy in time to avoid disaster [36]. In surgery it is often occasioned by stress, such as an operation on a life-threatening condition or an unexpected life-threatening complication during a planned elective intervention.

There is another interesting fact about anchoring. When we try to move away from the anchored figure and attempt to make adjustments, we are unable to move far enough and to make the necessary adjustment. Just like the ship that is attached to its anchor by a rope, we are tied to the starting point. These starting points may be unrelated to the issue. Daniel Kahneman, who was awarded the Nobel Prize in 2002, conducted an experiment in which he asked participants to estimate the percentage of African countries in the United Nations. Before the participants answered, they spun a specially numbered wheel of fortune, observed by the participant, and announced the number the wheel stopped at. The result was dramatic. The number from the wheel of fortune significantly influenced the estimates that participants made. Participants whose wheel number was 10 guessed on average 25 countries, and participants whose wheel number was 65 guessed on average 45 countries.

The particular danger of anchoring and adjustment is that we can easily think that we have taken account of its effect, when in fact we have not. People asked to estimate the percentage of African countries in the UN who started with the number 10 did adjust upwards – but only to an average of 25. Similarly, those who started with the number 65 adjusted downwards – but only to 45. It is also seen that anchoring has the effect of making us selective about information. We search for information that supports the anchored position and rejects the rest. When we have made a judgement, we tend to accept information that supports the judgement and reject other information.

How does this apply to surgical practice?

The following case example shows how a vascular surgeon anchored and adjusted the operative risk.

Case scenario

A 72-year-old woman with a recent stroke has resultant right hemiparesis that slowly improves over two days. Her CT scan shows a left hemispheric enhancing lesion with a diameter of 2cm. You have been called in as a vascular surgeon to consult on the case. What would you do?

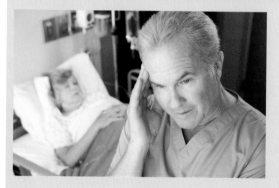

The first thing I would do is obtain a duplex scan of the neck and look for a source.

The Doppler shows a right-sided occlusion and a deep left-sided plaque with a 70% stenosis. Where would you go from there?

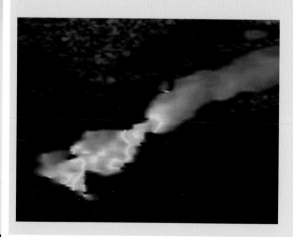

Continued

First, in addition to the duplex information, I want confirmation of the data with a CT angiogram. Then I would recommend an operation, after informed consent; this situation probably involves a higher stroke rate than the usual 2% or 3% because the patient has an occlusion on the contralateral side. And we know that an occlusion on the contralateral side increases the risk of a stroke and subsequent complications. Because of that, I'd quote a somewhat higher stroke complication rate, perhaps in the range of 5-10%, as opposed to 2-3%.

Surgeons need to respond appropriately to the risks of surgical procedures, knowing the probabilities of complications. But it is difficult to know the exact risk for a particular patient.

When justifying decisions – as in teaching, morbidity and mortality rounds, or when communicating with a patient – probability measures of the risk of a procedure are often heard. Here the vascular surgeon said the 72-year-old woman would have a stroke rate which "probably involves a higher stroke rate than the usual 2% or 3% because the patient has an occlusion on the contralateral side." He knows the numbers for the typical patient: 2-3%. And he knows that in her case the probability is higher: "We know that an occlusion on the contralateral side increases the risk of a stroke and subsequent complications." So he adjusts his estimate: "I'd quote a somewhat higher stroke complication rate, perhaps in the range of 5-10%, as opposed to 2-3%."

This probability adjustment has several interesting features. First, note that he is more uncertain about the adjusted probability, giving a range of 5% (from 5-10%) rather than a range of 1% (from 2-3%). Although the greater range may be more appropriate for the subset of patients (when the sample in any study has a smaller n, the estimate of the mean has greater uncertainty), this probably reflects the surgeon's uncertainty in his adjustment rather than the features of the studies from which he learned the numbers.

Second, in revising the probability for this particular patient, the surgeon has used a strategy of anchoring and adjustment – recalling a number that holds for a general class and then adjusting it to the characteristics of the particular individual. Here he recalled the stroke complication rate for carotid endarterectomies in general (2-3%) and adjusted it upward to 5-10% for the patient's particular situation (contralateral occlusion, age, history of stroke).

People often use this strategy. They anchor on a number that is quickly available and then adjust it. When making estimates for the first time, they may put too much weight on the initial anchor and adjust it insufficiently.

Overconfidence

Connected to anchoring is the overconfidence bias. The explanation for the overconfidence bias is the same as the explanation for the failure to adjust sufficiently from a starting point: anchoring.

Dr James Potchen did a study with radiologists [37]. More than a 100 radiologists were shown 60 chest X-rays and asked to give a diagnosis. One of the most interesting outcomes of the study was to compare the top 20 radiologists, who had an accuracy of nearly 95%, with the bottom 20, who had an accuracy of 75%. Most worrisome was the level of confidence each group had in its analysis. The radiologists who performed poorly were not only inaccurate, they were also very confident that they were right, when in fact they were wrong. The observers' lack of ability to discriminate normal from abnormal films did not necessarily diminish their confidence.

In our survey, we asked a question to a group of surgeons: in which deciles do you expect to fall in the distribution of surgical performance? Surgeons could claim the top 10%, the second 10%, and so on. Most surgeons are presumably well aware of bell distribution: half of the population would be in the top 50% and half in the bottom, and only 10% of the group can end up in the top deciles. Nevertheless, the results of the survey revealed a high degree of unrealistic self-appraisal among surgeons. Typically, less than 5% of the surgeons expected their performance to be below the medium (the 50th percent) and more than half expected to perform in one of the top two deciles. Invariably, the largest group of surgeons put themselves in the second decile. This could be seen as surgeons' modesty: they really think they belong in the top decile, but are too modest to say so!

Those who are overconfident tend to spend insufficient time accumulating evidence and synthesising it before action. They are more inclined to act on incomplete information. When overconfident people believe that their involvement might have a significant impact on outcomes (whether it actually does or not), they tend to strongly believe that the outcome will be positive. Overconfidence can combine badly with anchoring and availability bias described above, leading to an over-reliance on readily available (rather than valuable) information. It also results in significant errors of both omission and commission and results in unwarranted intervention, costly delays, or missed diagnoses. Overconfidence also plays a role in hindsight bias.

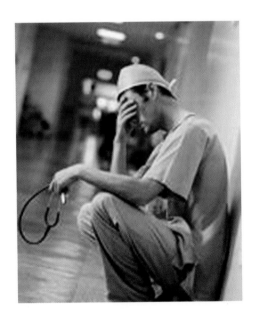

Confidence is important for success in a surgical career. Nothing that has been mentioned earlier should discourage you from believing in yourself and your ability to make good choices. Unfounded overconfidence, however, can get you into trouble. It is not what we don't know that gives us trouble – it is what we know that isn't so! Those individuals whose intellectual and interpersonal abilities are weakest are the most likely to overestimate their performance and ability. Apparently, as we become more knowledgeable about an issue, we are less likely to display overconfidence. Thus, overconfidence is more likely to surface when considering issues and problems that are outside of our area of expertise.

Here is a think-aloud of a confident surgeon.

Case scenario

A 65-year-old man is referred to you with a villous adenoma of the rectum located 6cm from the anal verge and encompassing one third to one half of the circumference of the rectum. Biopsy shows 'marked atypia'. What would you do?

After either further colonoscopy or barium enema to make sure that the patient has no lesion other than the one described at 6cm, I would take the patient to the operating room and, under general anaesthesia, widely dilate his anus and lower rectal sphincters. Then I would actually remove the lesion trans-anally, and with good margins.

As sometimes happens in villous adenomas with large lesions, a central carcinoma may be found in the middle of the villous adenoma. If this is proved to be true in the pathologic specimen, then further surgery may be required.

If there was actually an invasive carcinoma in the mid-portion of the lesion, I would return the patient to surgery, most likely for an abdomino-peritoneal procedure on a lesion this low.

A major feature of this surgeon's thinking about the case is sureness. Along with his recognition of the situation comes his choice of what to do, which is presented without hesitation and without consideration of alternatives. Of course the surgeon cannot predict what will happen – whether there will be a carcinoma in the centre of the adenoma, for example. But for each anticipated possible event, he has a clear response in mind.

One may question whether the surgeon's certainty brings with it a little rigidity, a reluctance to consider alternative approaches that may be better. Upon probing, of course, the surgeon knows very well the common alternatives and the arguments for and against. Having considered them adequately in the past, he does not need to bring up an awareness of the controversy each time he faces the situation.

Hindsight bias

There is a general tendency for us to believe (falsely) that we have accurately predicted the outcome of an event, after the outcome is actually known [38]. When something happens and we come to know what the outcome is, we seem to be good at concluding that this outcome was relatively obvious. For instance, a lot more people seem to have been sure about the inevitability of who would win the football match the day after the game.

The following scenario was given to five surgeons.

Case scenario

A 67-year-old male patient came to casualty with severe abdominal and back pain. He had been a smoker since the age of 25 and smoked 10 cigarettes every day. He enjoyed 2 to 3 glasses of whisky every night. His drug history included amlodipine, aspirin, simvastatin and diclofenac. On examination, he appeared pale and sweaty. His pulse rate was 110/min regular and his blood pressure was 100/60 mm Hg. His urine dipstick revealed blood 1+.

What is the likelihood of the following diagnoses?

1.	Ruptured abdominal aortic aneurysm	--------%
2.	Perforated duodenal ulcer	--------%
3.	Acute pancreatitis	--------%
4.	Renal colic	--------%
	Total	100 %

All the surgeons except one were told the actual diagnosis. They were asked to answer this scenario assuming that they were not aware of the 'actual' diagnosis. The tricky part was that every surgeon was told a different diagnosis. For example, the second surgeon was told that it was a perforated duodenal ulcer, while the fourth surgeon was told that it was a renal colic. Surgeons were asked to estimate the probability of the diagnoses, ignoring what they had been told about the 'actual' diagnosis. After they had marked their options, all five surgeons were asked for their estimates. It became apparent that they had estimated the diagnosis that they had been told was the actual diagnosis to be more likely. Consciously, they tried to ignore the diagnosis, and yet it affected their estimations. The surgeon who was told that a perforated duodenal ulcer was the 'actual' diagnosis rated that most likely, while the surgeon who was told renal colic rated that diagnosis as highly likely. Essentially, surgeons who had hindsight estimated the probability differently from surgeons who weren't aware of the diagnosis. Each inflated the probability of the diagnosis that he/she had been told. The thinking affected by hindsight bias was inappropriate, because the information about the actual diagnosis should not have affected their judgement [39].

What this indicates is that knowledge of the outcome focuses your attention on the information that is consistent with that outcome; that is, outcome knowledge draws

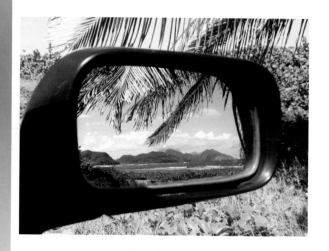

attention to the reasons why the diagnosis was predictable, but not to the reasons why alternative diagnoses were possible. The evidence that is consistent with the diagnosis is more easily recalled than facts that contradict the outcome.

Hindsight bias has an important clinical implication. Hindsight bias reduces our ability to learn from the past. It permits us to think that we were better at making predictions than we really are, and can result in us being more confident about the accuracy of future decisions than we have a right to be. If, for instance, your actual predictive accuracy is only 40%, but you think it is 90%, you are likely to become overconfident in your predictive skills. If surgeons assume that they would have predicted a clinical outcome, then they may fail to learn from a case. For example, unusual cases presented in meetings may seem predictable because of hindsight bias. You may conclude that you know this already and consequently fail to learn from the lessons illustrated by the case. We see this happening in morbidity and mortality rounds. Many errors appear transparent in hindsight. However, hindsight does not take into account the prevailing conditions at the time the decision was made.

Essentially, when we know the outcome, it significantly influences how we perceive past events. After an event has occurred, there is a tendency to exaggerate the likelihood that would have been assessed for the event before it occurred. Thus, when the events are viewed in hindsight, there is a tendency to attach a coherence of causality to them.

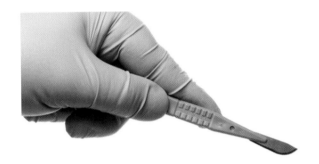

Error of commission

A surgeon is judged by the cases he refuses just as much as by the cases which he operates. Sometimes you face a dilemma of 'to operate or not to operate'. Taking the decision not to operate can be difficult for some surgeons. They tend to be activist, tempted to do something – sometimes, anything! By the nature of their personality, surgeons have a tendency towards action rather than inaction. But when this attitude is stretched too far, especially, without the surgeon being conscious and careful, the surgeon is at risk of committing a commission error. Someone who is known to be overconfident is likely to indulge in this commission-biased thinking. Sometimes, this commission bias is augmented by external pressures that require the surgeon to be seen as doing something. These pressures may be from the patient's family or the hospital management. Although superb operative skill wins admiration for surgeons, operative skill untempered by judgement can be dangerous, seducing surgeons into procedures that more prudent colleagues avoid.

If you remember the experience of Dr Groopman described earlier, Dr A showed what is called "commission bias" – that is, a tendency towards action rather than inaction. Commission error is more likely to happen with a surgeon whose ego is inflated, but it can also occur when a surgeon is desperate and gives in to the urge to 'do something'. This error is sometimes sparked by pressure from a patient and it takes considerable effort for a surgeon to resist. This bias takes on a different dimension when the financial aspects of the practice are involved.

In general, inaction is not at all what is expected from a surgeon, nor what a surgeon expects from himself; nevertheless, sometimes it is the best course. In deciding on the best strategy to manage localised prostate cancer, the outcome criteria include survival rates, quality of life, and treatment side effects, among others. If expectant management, i.e. watchful waiting, achieves better overall outcomes than prostatectomy, i.e. doing something, then expectant management is the optimal decision. Some decision analyses show this to be the case, although the issue is quite controversial. The fact that expectant management is a passive strategy and surgery an active strategy should not matter. Surgery does not give an extra advantage just because it involves doing something (as opposed to doing nothing). The fact that prostatectomy remains a frequent procedure suggests that surgeons' decisions may be influenced by commission bias.

This factor is involved in surgical procedures for asymptomatic patients [40]. Two assumptions underpin arguments for elective surgery when symptoms are mild or absent. The first is that the clinical problem targeted by the surgery will worsen over time, so that the patient will require the surgery eventually. The second is that delayed surgery will be more difficult or dangerous because of emergency circumstances or increased age. Data suggest that differences in the rate of transurethral resection among urologists can be explained by differences in the acceptance of these assumptions about surgery. However, careful analysis suggests that these assumptions are often wrong and that watchful waiting is a better option than elective surgery. Decision analysis shows that watchful waiting has fewer life risks than early prostate surgery when the patient has mild to moderate retention. Watchful waiting is also a better choice than prostatectomy for many categories of patients with localised prostate cancer. It is also a better choice than open surgery for asymptomatic gallstones. Careful risk-benefit analysis may reveal the advantage of this approach for many elective procedures. Other considerations weigh on the side of watchful waiting. The passage of time offers the chance of a technical breakthrough, for example, laparoscopic cholecystectomy instead of open cholecystectomy, and lithotripsy instead of kidney surgery. The data, however, show that the net results may be that the procedures are done far more often than would be justified. When randomised trials show no clear benefit of so-called preventive surgery, it may be better to follow a new rule of thumb for certain situations: do not operate when the patient can wait.

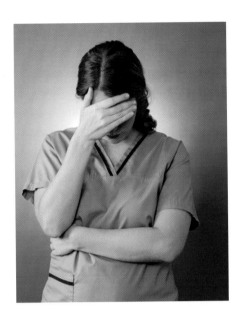

Error of omission

Some surgical procedures, on the other hand, may be under-utilised. Knee-replacement surgery may be such a case, considering the functional benefits that accrue to patients and the low rate of its use.

The opposite problem to commission bias is that some surgeons will avoid taking action in certain circumstances. Occasionally, they will just sit on a case in which they should intervene.

Consider the following case scenario.

Case scenario

Imagine that you are the parent of a one-year-old child.

You are living in an area where there is an endemic of 'xxx flu' with a fatality rate of 10 in 10,000.

A vaccination is available that could protect your child, but carries the risk of a fatal adverse reaction. The reported incidence of the fatal adverse reaction is 9 in 10,000.

Would you accept the vaccination for your child?

Logically, the relevant consequence in the decision is the risk of death. Any vaccine that lowers the risk of death from the 10-in-10,000 risk posed by the flu is preferable to the alternative of not vaccinating. Thus, it was expected that the majority of subjects would accept this vaccine, which has a 9 in 10,000 mortality risk. However, more than 50% of subjects declined the vaccine. They believed that the risk resulting from an omission (not vaccinating) is preferable to a death resulting from an act (vaccination) [41].

Omission bias is the tendency towards inaction or a reluctance to act. Inaction is preferred over action through fear of being held directly responsible for the outcome. Blame tends to be directed at the last person to have touched the patient. It has its origin in the idea that when a bad outcome occurs, blame will be more likely if you did something, rather than if you did not. It is preferable that an event is seen to happen naturally, rather than be directly attributed to the action of a surgeon. This tendency towards inaction may explain why passive euthanasia is preferred over active euthanasia, even though the end result is identical.

Multiple alternative errors

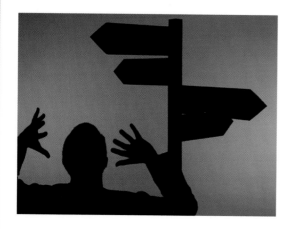

You have gone shopping to purchase an outfit. Consider that you are choosing an outfit out of the two selected in a shop. After comparing them, you decide to buy one. Now think of a situation in which you are choosing just one outfit out of five which you like. The choice of five outfits has increased the difficulty of making a decision. Obviously, it will take longer to make a decision in the second scenario. Not only will you take longer to decide, you are likely to revert back to choosing from the original two, or even decide to stay with the original.

The following research experiment was published in *JAMA* [42].

Case scenario A

Imagine that you are a GP and have been managing a 60-year-old gentleman suffering from osteoarthritis. You have tried various medications without success and have been considering referring the patient to an orthopaedic consultant for consideration of a hip replacement.

A few days before you are about to see this patient in the clinic, you become aware that there is a new medication available that you have not tried for this patient.

Which of the following actions would you take?

A) Referral to the orthopaedic consultant and not to start any new medication.

Or

B) Referral to the orthopaedic consultant and also start new medication.

Case scenario B

Imagine that you are a GP and have been managing a 60-year-old gentleman suffering from osteoarthritis. You have tried various medications without success and have been considering referring the patient to an orthopaedic consultant for consideration of a hip replacement.

A few days before you are about to see this patient in the clinic, you become aware that there are two new medications available that you have not tried for this patient (according to your information, both medications are equivalent in regard to their effects).

Continued

Which of the following actions would you take?

A) Referral to the orthopaedic consultant and not to start any new medication.

Or

B) Referral to the orthopaedic consultant and also start new medication A.

Or

C) Referral to the orthopaedic consultant and also start new medication B.

The typical observation was that, in the first scenario, about 50% of doctors chose the first option and the other 50% chose the second option. In the three-option condition, 90% of doctors chose the first option, the 'no medication' alternative. So while in the case of a two-option situation 50% chose to refer the patient to the orthopaedic surgeon without starting medication, in the three-option condition this proportion rose to 90%. Thus, the inclusion of alternative C increases the preference for alternative A.

The decision of referral was affected by an irrelevant factor – the availability of medications that had not been tried. The reason behind this decision was that in the three-option condition, the doctors found it difficult to explain why one selected medication A over medication B, or vice versa. This decision conflict was avoided by selecting the default option A: referring the patient to an orthopaedic surgeon without starting new medication, making this option particularly attractive. In the two-option condition, there is no such decision conflict between two similar options that can be resolved by selecting the third.

Biases induced by adding additional choice alternatives are relevant to current surgical practice, where new treatments or procedures frequently become available. While one might think that additional options for treatment would likely improve medical care, the studies reviewed in this section suggest that additional options may alter decisions in ways that are not necessarily an improvement.

In a clinical situation, doctors feel relatively comfortable about choosing between two alternatives. However, if options expand, they experience difficulty with the additional choices and tend to fall back on the status quo. Paradoxically, it appears that instead of the new alternatives inviting a wider range of choice, the uncertainty and conflicts drive the decision maker back to more conservative behaviour.

As a surgeon, you are used to a particular prosthesis for knee replacement. You later receive information about a new prosthesis – let's say Type B – which appears to be a reasonable alternative to the one that you are using (Type A). You are inclined to consider this new Type B prosthesis, which might offer some benefits over Type A. While you are in the process of exploring that option, you are told that a third prosthesis, Type C, has entered into the market, which has some advantages over the prosthesis you are currently using. The reasonable approach would be to consider both these new prostheses and evaluate them for their efficacy. However, the multiple alternative bias predicts that some of you would tend to revert to prosthesis A, because multiple choices generate conflict and uncertainty. This is also a variant of 'status quo' bias – in other words, preferring the known to the unknown. But the multiple alternative biases go a little further than that in creating an irrational inertia against optimising choice among competing alternatives. Thus, situations that create multiple alternatives can lead to irrational decision-making and may in fact result in suboptimal treatment.

Aggregate bias

Mike, a registrar in orthopaedics, was asked to see a patient with a minor ankle injury. He examined the patient and concluded that the patient had just sprained the muscles and there was no reason to believe that he had any fracture. As per the hospital protocol, Mike went through the 'Ottawa ankle rule' protocol, which confirmed that the patient did not need any further investigation. As he was about to send the patient home, he asked the patient to come back and ordered an X-ray of his ankle. Why did he change his mind and order an X-ray that he had previously thought was unnecessary? There was no reason to believe that Mike obtained any additional clinical information that made him change his plan. Even the hospital protocol he was supposed to follow did not indicate that the patient needed any further investigation. What could explain Mike's change of heart? The answer is 'aggregate bias' [43].

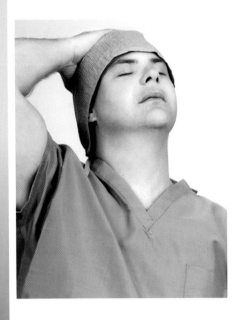

Mike's thinking was hampered by this bias, which could be blamed for his change of heart. Aggregate bias is one of the reasons why surgeons do not follow guidelines in some cases. When your thinking is influenced by this bias you treat the patient differently to the general acceptable norm. If Mike had been asked to explain his decision, he would have defended it by saying something like, "Oh, this patient's presentation is not typical; he is not an average patient. That's why..." If he had been challenged further as to why he thought that the patient was unusual, he would not have been able to justify his thinking satisfactorily. Thus, in cases of aggregate bias, you (wrongly) think that the patient's presentation is atypical when actually it is not; you unnecessarily put the patient in the 'unusual' or atypical category. Just to make it clear, if there is any clinical feature that causes you to suspect that the case is atypical, that should not be a problem – the problem occurs when you start thinking that this is an atypical case even though there are no clinical grounds for your suspicion. This kind of thinking affects compliance with evidence-based guidelines. Although you are well aware of the guideline, you think that this patient would not be eligible for the criteria of the guideline, when in actuality he would have been. As a consequence of this thinking error, a patient may be deprived of the procedure that he deserves, or may be subjected to unnecessary investigations or intervention.

Search-satisfying error

If you remember the case of Dr Jerome Groopman, you may recollect that he consulted a second orthopaedic surgeon, Dr B. As soon as Dr B saw the MRI, he saw a hairline fracture and cysts in the scaphoid and a tiny cyst in another bone. He concluded that he had found out the cause of the patient's symptom and advised surgery. The cognitive error Dr B made is called the 'satisfaction of search'. This is the tendency to stop searching for a diagnosis once you find something. The patient has a symptom that the surgeon needs to explain. As he searches for the explanation, he finds something wrong in the physical examination or in the investigation. That is what happened when Dr B jumped on the bone cysts in the MRI scan. The problem is that there may be more than one thing to be found.

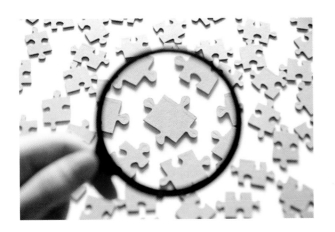

Search-satisfying is the tendency to call off a search once something is found. If we lose an object in everyday life, we start looking for it and the search begins. Consequently, the search will be called off once the object we lost has been found. However, in a clinical set-up, the situation is different. There may often be more than one thing to be found. We are not always sure what it looks like, and we do not always know where to look. If a fracture is found, there may be a second or third fracture, or radiographic signs of soft-tissue injury; there may be more than one foreign body in the wound. The patient may have more than one diagnosis. In all of these cases, satisfying one's self that the surgery is over once something has been found will be erroneous.

This satisfaction-of-search tendency is seen in our everyday lives as well. Say you are getting ready to leave the house to catch a flight and you are running late. You look for your passport but it is not in the drawer where you usually leave it. You begin to panic. You start looking for it frantically and find it on the night table. You feel relieved that you have found the passport and put it in your pocket. Now you will be able to catch the flight. After putting the passport in your pocket, walking out of your house, closing the door and approaching your car, you realise that you are missing your car keys. You have also closed the front door and can't get back in without your house key, which is on the same key-ring as the car keys. You were so pleased about finding your passport that your mind shut down and you didn't consider what else was missing.

Finding something may be satisfactory, but not finding everything is sub-optimal. An additional problem in the case of surgery is that the surgeon may not have been searching in the right place, in which case the search will be called off once it appears that there is nothing to be found. Similarly, calling off the search when something has been found can lead to significant further findings being missed. For example, significant traumatic injuries rarely occur in isolation. There will usually be other findings, but searching in the wrong place will result in nothing being found.

Do you know which fracture is missed most frequently?

The answer is – the second fracture.

Sunk-cost bias

A lot of us get sucked in by a sunk cost when making decisions. For example, have you ever had anyone tell you that they are unhappy in their relationship? If you ask that person why he or she doesn't move on, the answer is invariably something like, "Because I have already put so much time into it." Do you know anybody who has stayed through a movie he could not bear to watch rather than walk out, just because he had paid £7 to see it?

A study of 8,000 surgeons was conducted in which they were asked questions regarding their job satisfaction [44]. A significant proportion (around 40%) of surgeons expressed dissatisfaction with their surgical career. Two of the questions were:

- Would you ask your child to be a surgeon?

- If the clock was turned back and you were given the opportunity to choose your career again, would you choose the same career?

In their replies, 50% of surgeons said that they would not recommend a surgical career to their children. However, when it came to their own choice, 75% said that they would do it again. It is interesting that 25% of surgeons won't recommend the job to their children but would happily do it themselves again. There are various explanations for this disparity. One of the explanations is 'sunk-cost bias'. Because surgeons have invested so much of their time and energy in their surgical career, they feel obliged to continue it, in spite of the unhappiness involved.

The common thread running through these examples is the consideration of sunk cost. When a person is taken in by the concept of sunk cost, they forget that the decision should be based only on future consequences. The decision you make today can only influence the future. No current decision can correct the past.

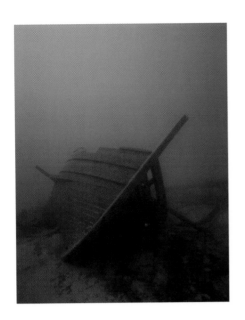

Why do so many of us act irrationally when it comes to ignoring past expenditure of time, money or effort? Why do we fixate on the past rather than on the future? Because ignoring sunk cost can make us look indecisive, and wasteful [45], we want to avoid admitting that an earlier decision was a mistake. "I have invested too much to quit now" is a phrase many of us have used too often. We also want to appear consistent. This is because consistency is a key element of rationality.

Conclusion

In an article entitled, 'The importance of cognitive errors in diagnosis and strategies to minimize them', Pat Croskerry argues that the cognitive revolution in psychology that took place over the previous 30 years gave rise to an extensive, empirical literature on cognitive biases in decision-making [46]. But this advance has been ponderously slow to enter medicine. Some people have clung to the old models of decision-making, which have little practical application in the real world. What is needed instead is the application of 'flesh and blood' decision-making. If we accept the pervasiveness and predictability of biases that underline cognitive error, then we are obliged to search for effective de-biasing techniques. Despite the prevailing pessimism, it has been demonstrated that, by using a variety of strategies, we would be able to overcome a number of specific biases. It appears that there are indeed cognitive pills for cognitive ills, which makes intuitive sense. The first step is to overcome the bias against overcoming the bias.

Key points

◆ Most of the day-to-day decisions involve using heuristics.

◆ Although effective most of the time, it creates biases that ultimately affect our judgement.

◆ To improve our decision-making, the first step we need to take is to become aware of these biases and monitor their effect on our thinking.

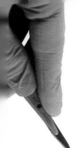

Chapter 5

Intuition – does it makes any sense?

Here is a story from the first Gulf War in 1991, when coalition battleships were deployed off the Kuwaiti coast [47]. Lieutenant Commander Michael Riley was monitoring the radar screens on board the HMS Gloucester, a British battleship. The ship was responsible for protecting the coalition fleet. At 5 o'clock in the morning, he noticed a radar blip off the Kuwaiti coast. A quick calculation of its trajectory had it heading for the convoy. Although Riley had been staring at similar blips all night long, there was something about this radar trace that immediately made him suspicious. He couldn't explain why, but the blinking green dot on the screen filled him with apprehension. He continued to observe the incoming blip for another 40 seconds as it slowly honed in on the USS Missouri, an American battleship. It was approaching the American ship at more than 500 miles per hour. If Riley was going to shoot down the target – if he was going to act on his fear – then he needed to respond right away. If Riley did not move immediately, it would be too late. The USS Missouri would be sunk and Riley would have stood by and watched it happen.

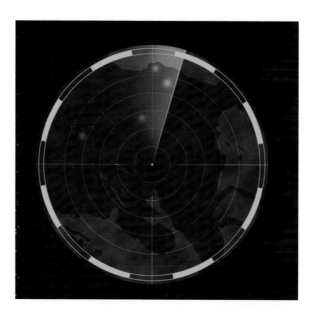

But Riley had a problem. The radar blip was located in airspace that was frequently used by American A6 fighter jets. The blip was travelling at the same speed as the fighter jets. It looked exactly like an A6 on the radar screen. To make matters even more complicated, the A6 pilots had gotten into the habit of turning off their electronic identification on their return flights. As a result, the radar crew on board the HMS Gloucester had no way of contacting them.

The target was moving fast. Riley issued the order to fire; two Sea Dart surface-to-air missiles were launched. Soon an explosion echoed over the ocean. The captain of the HMS Gloucester asked Riley how he could be sure he had fired at an Iraqi missile and not an American fighter jet. Riley said: "I just knew."

I am sure you have had similar experiences many times. Not of firing a missile, but of the feeling of, "I just knew." There are many actions surgeons take that they find difficult to explain. In the early days of your training, you might have observed an experienced surgeon making a diagnosis of a very complex case just by history and examination. If you had asked him how he reached his decision, he might have said, "I just knew." Some call it experience, while others say it is intuition. Decision science calls it 'system 1 thinking'.

The next four hours were the longest of Riley's life. If he had shot down an A6, then he had killed two innocent pilots, and his career was over. After a four-hour wait, the captain of the HMS Gloucester was informed that the radar blip was, in fact, a Silkworm missile, and not an American fighter jet. Riley had single-handedly saved a battleship.

After the war was over, British naval officers analysed the events preceding Riley's decision to fire the Sea Dart missiles. They concluded that, with the information available to Lieutenant Commander Riley, it was impossible for him to distinguish between the Silkworm and a friendly A6. Although Riley had made the correct decision, he could just as easily have been shooting down an American fighter jet. His risky gamble paid off, but it had still been a gamble.

That, at least, was the official version of events until Gary Klein, a cognitive psychologist, got involved. He proved that it was nothing like a gamble. Gary soon realised that Riley had gotten used to seeing very consistent blip patterns when A6s returned from their bombing sorties. The planes typically became visible after a single radar sweep. Klein analysed the radar tapes from the predawn missile attack. He replayed those fateful 40 seconds over and over again, searching for any differences between Riley's experience of A6s returning from their sorties and his experience of the Silkworm blip. Klein suddenly saw the discrepancy. It was subtle, but crystal clear. He could finally explain Riley's thought process. The secret was timing. Unlike the A6, the Silkworm did not appear off the coast right away. Because it travelled at such a low altitude – nearly 2,000 feet below an A6 – the signal of the missile was initially masked by ground interference. As a result, it was not visible until the third radar sweep, which was eight seconds after an A6 would have appeared. Riley was unconsciously evaluating the altitude of the blip, even if he did not know he was.

This is why Riley got the chills when he stared at the Iraqi missile on his radar screen. There was something strange about the radar blip. It did not feel like an A6. Although Riley could not explain why he felt so scared, he knew that something scary was happening. This blip needed to be shot down.

There are two reasons for mentioning this story here: firstly, to get interesting accounts of intuitive decision-making; and, secondly, to show how other professionals are taking intuitive decision-making seriously. The military has taken intuitive decision-making to a formal level. The military has incorporated intuitive decision-making in its training programme. This has been a massive change for an organisation that is run on strict rules and procedures.

Although it has been known for a long time that surgeons use intuitive thinking, it has not been given serious consideration. We hardly know anything about it. If we have any problems due to the process of intuitive thinking, isn't it a good idea to know some basic things about it?

First of all, why should we be bothered about intuition?

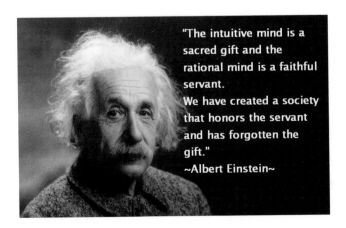

"The intuitive mind is a sacred gift and the rational mind is a faithful servant.
We have created a society that honors the servant and has forgotten the gift."
~Albert Einstein~

We need to reclaim the gift. Conventional methods of surgical practice and surgical training are becoming outdated. Unless we make conscious efforts to sharpen our intuitive skills, we may not be able to perform effectively and efficiently. Guidelines and protocols have a certain place in management. They can be useful for run-of-the-mill diagnoses and treatment. But they quickly fall apart when you need to think outside the box, and when symptoms are vague or multiple and the investigations are inconclusive. To manage these kinds of cases, you need discerning thinking. Protocols discourage surgeons from thinking independently and creatively. Instead of expanding clinicians' thinking, they can restrain it. Imagine you are performing an endoscopy. You feel a little resistance while inserting the scope. A few seconds later, an enormous gush of blood blows out of the scope! You are in trouble. No guideline, no protocol, can help you in this situation. The only thing that can save you is your intuition.

There are a lot of misconceptions about intuition. According to Benner, "...intuition is the black-market version of the knowledge" [48]. There are individuals who are ignorant and intolerant towards the idea of intuitive thinking. They may not realise the disadvantage they incur due to their attitude. They may not be aware; they may not trust intuition, but they can't live without it. Unfortunately, we have not taken a scientific approach towards this wonderful faculty. Similar to other scientific developments, cognitive science has progressed over the last few years. It would be unwise to remain fixated on the traditional view of intuition.

So let's start with a basic question: what is intuition? To get the answer, think about the times when you had a sense about something, even though you couldn't quite explain it. What is it that sets off the alarm bells inside your head when apparently the case appears to be just a routine one? It is an intuition, built up through repeated experiences that you have unconsciously linked together to form a pattern. That's how we have hunches about what is really going on and about what we should do.

The more patterns we learn, the easier it is to match a new situation to one of the patterns in your reservoir. When a new situation occurs, we recognise the situation as familiar by matching it to a pattern we have encountered in the past. Once we recognise a pattern, we gain a sense of situation: we know what cues are going to be important and need to be monitored. We have a sense of what to expect next. And the patterns include routines for responding. If we see a situation as typical, then we can recognise the typical ways to react.

The following think-aloud will illustrate intuition in a surgical context. Here, a consultant general surgeon is asked to put across his views about the management of a patient.

Case scenario

A 16-year-old girl reports right lower-quadrant (RLQ) pain for 6 hours and mild RLQ tenderness. Her temperature is 37°C and there is no nausea or vomiting. She is in the mid-cycle of her menstrual period. The WBC count is 7,800 with no shift. What are your thoughts?

You are always worried about appendicitis, but it's early in the course of events. People usually don't have to worry about a ruptured appendix for 24-36 hours. If you don't think she has surgical indications, it's probably safe to watch her. It sounds like she probably has mittelschmerz because she is mid-cycle in her period; assuming she is not on birth-control pills. You need to know if she is hungry or not, and if she typically has such pain during her cycle. You also need to do a pelvic exam. I wouldn't operate on her at this point.

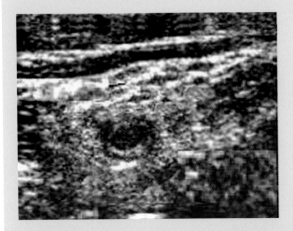

An ultrasound of the pelvis shows a slight amount of fluid in the cul-de-sac but is otherwise normal.

Same thing – she could have a ruptured cyst which wasn't identified on the ultrasound.

The pain persists overnight. Tenderness in the RLQ persists. Laparoscopy is performed by the on-call surgeon. The tubes, ovaries, and appendix are normal. What would you do in this situation?

The appendix, tubes, and ovaries are normal. I would probably do a laparoscopic appendectomy while I was there, but I would not do anything further.

Continued

What triggers an operation for possible appendicitis? What does not trigger it?

I think the single most important thing is how tender the patient is over the appendix, in association with a compatible history. What does not trigger me to operate on appendicitis? Early in the course, less than 6 hours, less than 24 hours, I am not as worried. White blood cell counts don't help me very much. Patients who are hungry usually don't have appendicitis. A lot of people say they are hungry, but I think only once in my life have I had a patient with appendicitis who wanted to go to McDonald's for a Big Mac and fries, which is my standard question. They frequently say, "Sure, I'm hungry," and I say, "You want a Big Mac and fries at McDonald's?" and they go, "Uh, I don't think so." It's a rare patient who is hungry. I am inclined not to jump on them if it's particularly early in the course and the situation is confusing. But the single most important determining factor is how tender the patient is over the appendix. In a patient with localised tenderness and significant guarding who is over 24 hours out, I simply take out the appendix. It's a clinical decision.

This case illustrates how we use intuition in a routine surgical case. This surgeon's thoughts concerning whether to operate for suspected appendicitis are an example of intuitive judgement. The surgeon pays attention to several factors simultaneously – amount and location of tenderness, duration of symptoms, appetite – and bases the decision on them. He cannot verbalise the rules governing the decision precisely. Judgements of this type have several features that differentiate them from analytical thinking. First, the result of the judgement is one of three possible actions: send the patient home, wait and see what develops, or operate. Second, several features have a bearing on the judgement, such as the patient's sex, age, and weight. Also relevant are features of the present illness, such as location, intensity, and quality of the right lower-quadrant pain, as well as the patient's appetite. But it is not just the current state of these variables that is important: the surgeon also pays attention to how they have varied over the past few hours and days. These variables actually make the decision even simpler, for they allow the surgeon to focus on just two actions: send home versus wait or wait versus operate. Of course, as the situation changes, the surgeon may focus on a different pair of options, but at any one moment the decision is simply between two alternatives. A third feature of such judgements is that the experts do not know exactly how they make them. They can say sensible things about each feature, such as, "If the patient has an appetite, it is probably not appendicitis," but they cannot say how the various features are combined into their overall sense of whether they should operate.

Intuition is the way we translate our experiences into decisions. It is that ability to make decisions by using patterns to recognise what is going on in a situation and to recognise the typical action plan with which to react. Once an experienced intuitive decision-maker sees the pattern, any decision they have to make is usually obvious.

A pattern is a set of features that usually chunk together so that if you see a few of the features you can expect to find the others. When you notice a pattern, you have a sense of familiarity – yes, I have seen it before! As we work in our particular professional field, we accumulate experiences and build up a reservoir of recognised patterns. The more patterns and action plans we have available, the more expertise we have, and the easier it is to make decisions. Without the repertoire of patterns and action scripts, we would have to painstakingly think out every situation from scratch. Because pattern matching can take place in an instant, and without conscious thought, we are not aware of how we arrived at an intuitive judgement. That is why it often seems mysterious to us. Even if the situation isn't exactly the same as anything we have seen before, we can recognise similarities with past events and so we automatically know what to do, without having to deliberately think out the options. We have a sense of what will work and what won't.

The other, rather interesting, way to describe intuition is to say, it's a joke. Yes, you read it correctly: intuition is a joke. To be specific, it is like a joke. When you listen to a joke, you find it funny. The joke is funny only if you get it. And you get it instantly, like a flash. If you don't get the joke and if somebody explains it you, it loses the punch and the fun. The instant appreciation of a joke is equivalent to instant recognition by intuition. Just as some people lack a sense of humour, some people do not develop an intuitive sense. On the other hand, like some 'very funny' people, some have a strong intuitive sense. To complete the analogy, for you to get the joke you need to know the background and context of the joke. The same is true of intuition. You need to know the context of a clinical situation to make an intuitive decision.

Here is another case given to a neurosurgeon.

Case scenario

You have gone to see a football match at your local club. A 16-year-old football player becomes unconscious for 30 seconds, and then walks to the sidelines. You are called to the sidelines to see him. How would you examine him? What would you do?

I am assuming that the mechanism was not a fall while he was running for a pass by himself. That suggests subarachnoid haemorrhage, like a spontaneous bleed into a brain tumour, although such a mechanism is unlikely in a 16-year-old. It's not going to be diffuse axonal injury for two reasons: number one, he got up and walked to the sidelines; and the second reason is that diffuse axonal injury is a big mechanism.

So it isn't going to be a diffuse axonal injury, because the mechanism is not right. The mechanism is right for a contusion of the brain. The chance of a subdural haematoma is very small, because firstly, the mechanism is not right, and second, he's too young. The possibility of an epidural haematoma is also very small. You need a skull fracture. So you're probably looking at a contusion, possibly as minor as a concussion.

How would you manage him?

I'd look at three things: level of consciousness, pupillary exam, and best motor response.

He is awake and alert. The pupillary exam is normal. The motor exam is normal as well; he can jog up and down the field.

He sits out for at least 5 or 6 minutes. Has his neurological exam changed?

No, it has not changed.

Then the question is, "Is he laying down any new information? Does he know what the score is?"

Continued

He is a little fuzzy on what happened to him.

Then he doesn't go back in.

He doesn't go back in the game? Does he go to the hospital?

If he gets any worse, he goes to the hospital immediately. He should only get better from the moment of impact, not worse.

You examine him and you talk to him. He is really fuzzy and doesn't know what is going on. He complains of a mild headache. You send him to the hospital. Does he have to have a CT scan?

When he gets to the hospital, has he gotten any worse?

He still has retrograde amnesia and keeps repeating the same question: "What happened to me? What happened to me?" But beyond that he is okay.

In that case, he would get a CT scan.

I notice you didn't look in his fundi.

No. That wastes time.

Why? Doesn't it help you?

No. You know what his neurological exam is. You know exactly how his whole brain is functioning.

You don't need a reflex hammer?

I don't need a reflex hammer. You see how you have to take the situation of your practice into account.

Pattern recognition

Have you noticed in this think-aloud how the neurosurgeon recognised and focused on key elements of the case? His thinking is efficient for various reasons. In addition to the knowledge, which is well organised for rapid access, the surgeon also knows what is important and can focus on the key elements of the case.

Thus, when initially engaged in pattern recognition, the surgeon knows to pay attention to the mechanism of the injury – a tackle involves more force than a spontaneous bleed into a brain tumour, but less than would produce a diffuse axonal injury. Large numbers of possibilities are eliminated through the use of one, highly diagnostic cue.

Later, he focuses on any changes in the football player's ability to think. Because the boy can reveal his state of consciousness, any more detailed neurological exam would be redundant. Any deterioration in his awareness would make the surgeon send him to the hospital.

Expert clinicians condense a case into manageable form, focusing on one or two pivotal findings. Success with this strategy depends, of course, on being able to judge which of many possible features of the case to focus on.

Gary Klein is a decision scientist who worked with the British Navy in relation to the incident during the Gulf War. He has worked with health professionals, military personnel and fire-fighters, studying decision-making processes in the workplace. Here is a case example from a study of decision-making he conducted with fire-fighters and has written a book, *Power of Intuition* [49].

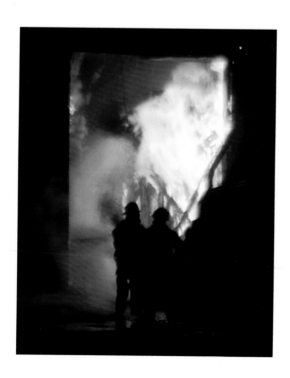

Case scenario

The fire brigade was called to manage a fire in the basement of a four-storey building. When the fire-fighters arrived, they did not see anything. The commander went to the basement and saw flames spreading up the laundry chute. For him it was a simple vertical fire. Since there was no sign of smoke, he thought the fire must just be starting. The way to tackle a vertical fire is to get above it and spray water down. So the commander sent one crew up to the first floor and another to the second. Both came back saying the fire had gotten past them. The commander realised that the fire had gone straight up to the fourth floor. Since there was no smoke when the fire brigade arrived just a minute earlier, this must have only just happened. It was obvious to him that the chance to put out the fire quickly had gone. He needed to change the strategy to search and rescue, and to get everyone out of the building.

This was a typical incident for Gary to study in terms of the fire-fighters' decision-making. He chose to study fire-fighters because, like surgeons, fire-fighters' work involves critical decision-making. Whatever he describes in relation to the way fire-fighters go about their work is similar to your own thinking when you come across a critical clinical situation. Gary was expecting to see hard decision-making activity. But during incidents like this one, he often used to wonder, "where was the decision?" The commander saw a vertical fire and knew just what to do. But, in an instant, that decision was no longer relevant because the fire had spread. The commander still knew exactly what to do in this changed situation. He never seemed to decide anything. The research team tried hard to find out how the commanders used two options and used analytical reasoning. They wanted to see how the commanders wrestled with choices. Surprisingly, none of these things happened. Gary was puzzled as to how the commanders could evaluate an option without comparing it to any others. He soon realised that the commanders did not have to compare options. They could come up with a good course of action from the start. Even when faced with a complex situation, the commanders could see it as familiar and knew how to react. The commanders' secret was that their experience let them see a situation, so they knew the typical course of action right away. Their experience let them identify a reasonable action as the first one they considered, so they did not bother thinking about others. The whole thing reminds me of a surgeon who would say, "We surgeons just act; we don't waste time in thinking. We tend to dive into the swamp and look around for alligators, while physicians analyse the swamp of water for its nutrient content to see if the water will support life. We are plungers; they are planners."

In some cases that Gary Klein studied, the fire-fighters did look at several options, yet they never compared them. The fire-fighter thought of each option one at a time, evaluated each in turn, rejected it and turned to the next rescue technique. This strategy is called the singular evaluation approach, to distinguish it from comparative evaluation. Distinguishing between comparative and singular evaluation is not difficult. When you order from a menu in a restaurant, you probably compare the different items to find the one you want the most. You are performing a comparative evaluation because you're trying to see if one item seems tastier than the others. In contrast, if you are in an unfamiliar town and you notice that your car is low on petrol, you start searching for a petrol pump and stop at the first reasonable place you find. You do not need the best petrol pump in the town.

Gary realised that a fire commander could judge a situation as typical and knew what to do. If their first choice did not work out, they might consider others – not to find the best, but to find the first one that works. But then there was a second puzzle. If the commanders did not compare options, how did they know that a course of action was any good?

To evaluate a course of action, the commander imagined himself carrying it out. He used the technique of mental simulation or visualisation, running the action through his mind. If he spotted a potential problem, he moved on to the next option and the next, until he found one that seemed to work.

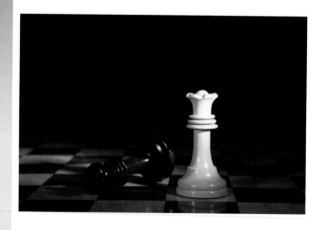

This is very similar to the chess grandmasters choosing their move in a game of chess; each move should be as strong as possible. This is particularly true at the grandmaster level, where even one or two slack moves – not blunders, but simply weak moves – can lead to defeat. Therefore, we would expect that chess grandmasters would be using all the methods developed by the decision scientist. They do not. The idea of generating a set of options and evaluating them misses the intuitive strength of chess grandmasters. The grandmasters do want to find the best possible move, and they do examine more than one move, but the way they do this tells us a lot. They use their intuition to recognise the promising moves that they should examine more closely. They shift to an analytic mode by looking at the moves as they will play out in the context of the game, and rely on their ability to mentally simulate what will happen if they play a move. In the course of these mental simulations, some of the moves drop out because they are found to contain weaknesses. By the end of their mental simulations, the grandmasters are usually only left with a single move that they consider playable. In the cases where they have two or more moves that they consider playable, the choice seems to depend on an intuitive sense of how they felt about the board position as they were doing the mental simulations. The move that triggers the most positive 'gut feeling' is chosen. Thus, although grandmasters are ferociously trying to find the best choice, they are not using analytical methods. If this type of strategy is good enough for chess grandmasters, it should be good enough for surgeons as well.

Visualisation in surgical decision-making

Case scenario

A 30-year-old woman had a laparoscopic cholecystectomy for acute cholecystitis six weeks previously. She is now jaundiced with a bilirubin of 14μmol/L and alkaline phosphates of 350IU/L. AST and ALT levels are normal. What are your thoughts? What work-up would you use?

You would have to be concerned that you have either injured her common bile duct or left behind a stone in the bile duct. She needs an endoscopic retrograde cholangio-pancreatography (ERCP) as the next step, which would be diagnostic and potentially therapeutic.

They are unable to do an ERCP. What will you do now?

I would do a transhepatic cholangiogram in an attempt to define where the problem was. Then she would have to have an operation.

A percutaneous transhepatic cholangiogram shows several clips at the area of the cystic duct stump with a 0.5cm narrowing of the common duct adjacent to the clips. What would you do?

I am trying to visualise what you just told me. You would have to assume a duct injury. I think I would operate on the patient.

Continued

Describe what you would do in the operation.

You have to figure out what is wrong. The patient has developed a stricture. You probably have a common duct injury from the procedure itself. It may be as simple as the fact that you put the clips too close to the common bile duct, and you may be able to alleviate the problem by removing them and closing over the cystic duct. If the duct has been significantly injured like cut in two, it will have to be repaired, probably with a Roux-en-Y choledochojejunostomy as opposed to a direct repair by putting the two ends of the duct together. It's hard for me to visualise the problem, but you have to find out what's wrong, and you have to operate to do it. Then you have to make the appropriate repair.

Given a description of postoperative complications, the surgeon tries to visualise what went wrong. He would prefer ERCP, with its superior visualisation and the possibility of inserting instruments, over the static image of the cholangiogram. If it were his own operation, he also might "rewind the video tape," recalling the operation to see if any details of the procedure could explain what is happening now. Given a verbal description of the results of the cholangiogram, the surgeon needs time to visualise them, to create an image of the patient's organs after the cholecystectomy. Knowledge from a variety of sources goes into this visualisation: knowledge of the normal anatomy of the organs, the disease that led to the original operation and the typical efficacy of that operation, and the procedures used when the gallbladder is removed via a laparoscope, as opposed to an open operation. It takes time to construct a full visualisation. This is not just due to the fact that the surgeon was not offered an X-ray, for it takes time to interpret an X-ray image too. The surgeon did not get a complete picture of exactly what had happened, but could assume it was a duct injury and that an operation is therefore necessary.

Before Gary Klein started the study, he believed that novices impulsively jumped at the first option they could think of, whereas experts carefully deliberated about the merits of different courses of action. Now it seemed that it was the experts who could generate a single course of action, while novices needed to compare different approaches. It wasn't the case that the fire-fighters never deliberated about options. They did, though only very occasionally – approximately less than 20% of the time.

Once, Gary encountered the following incident.

Case scenario

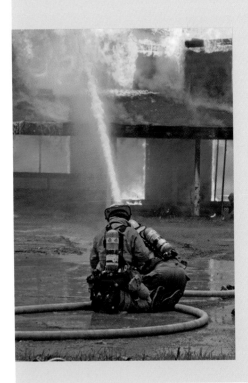

It was a simple house fire in a one-storey house. The fire was in the back, in the kitchen area. The commander led his hose screw into the back of the house to spray water on the fire, but the fire just roared back at them. "Odd," he thought. They tried dousing it again and got the same results. Then the commander started to feel as if something was not right. He didn't have any clue; he just didn't feel right about being in the house, so he ordered his men out of the house. As soon as his men left the house, the floor on which they had been standing collapsed. Had they still been inside, all of them would have plunged into the fire below.

When Gary Klein spoke to the commander after the incident, he was not able to give an explanation as to why he decided to pull out. "I just did," was his answer. Does it sound like the answer we hear from surgeons? In this case, further exploration revealed some interesting facts. The commander did not suspect that the seat of the fire was in the basement, directly underneath the living room where he and his men were standing, when he gave his order to evacuate. But he was already wondering why the fire did not react as expected. The living room was hotter than he would have expected for a small fire in the kitchen. It was a very quiet fire. Fires are noisy, and for a fire with this much heat he would have expected a great deal of noise. Thus the whole pattern did not seem right and he realised he did not quite know what was going on. That was why he ordered his men out of the building. With hindsight, the reason for the mismatch was clear. Because the fire was under him and not in the kitchen, it was not affected by his crew's attack. The rising heat was much greater than he had expected and the floor acted like a baffle to muffle the noise, resulting in a hot but quiet environment.

This incident helps to understand how we make decisions by recognising when an atypical situation is developing. In this case, the events were not typical, and the commander's reaction was to pull back. This shows us what happens when the pattern does not fit together. The commander's experience had provided him with a set of patterns. He was accustomed to sizing up a situation by having it match one of these patterns. He may not have been able to describe its features, but he was relying on the pattern-matching process to let him feel comfortable that he had the situation scoped out. Nevertheless, he did not seem to be aware of how he was using his experience because he was not doing it consciously. He could see what was going on in front of his eyes but not what was going on behind them.

This is one basis for what we call intuition: recognising things without knowing how we do the recognising. We size the situation up and immediately know how to proceed: which goals to pursue, what to expect, and how to respond. We are drawn to certain clues and not others because of our situation awareness; this must happen all the time. Let us see another surgical example.

Decisions depend on pattern recognition

Case scenario

A 55-year-old man presents with gross melaena. Four units of blood are required to restore his blood pressure to normal. Endoscopy demonstrates a posterior duodenal ulcer with an oozing vessel in the base. What are your thoughts?

If the duodenum is terribly scarred and you had to do a resection to get at it, I would insert a tube duodenostomy and close it. This procedure always works to keep you out of trouble in an emergency situation.

On the fifth postoperative day the patient is jaundiced with a bilirubin of 8μmol/L and an alkaline phosphatase of 300IU/L; the other liver enzymes are normal. What would you do?

The patient needs an endoscopic retrograde cholangio-pancreatography (ERCP) or a percutaneous transhepatic cholangiogram to make sure that I did not injure his common bile duct with my sutures. I would think back over exactly what I did, suture wise, at the operation and see if I feasibly could have put a suture around the common duct.

Continued

On the seventh postoperative day, the patient vomits a large amount of blood. What would you do?

I would repeat the endoscopy if at all possible. The patient could be bleeding from the suture line. I would keep in mind that the gastroenterologist can sometimes zap something and save the patient an operation. I would re-operate if they couldn't figure it out or if he was bleeding profusely.

The surgeon rapidly recognises and responds to the situation. The elements of good decisions are present in these responses, although it is not easy to see them because the responses take place so quickly.

To make good decisions, one must know the options. In this think-aloud, the surgeon comes up with appropriate options. If the situations were different, different options would come to mind. One of the features of the human memory is that ideas come to mind when they are likely to be needed.

The surgeon must also know what can happen. Examples in the think-aloud include the surgeon's comment on the tube duodenostomy, that it can "keep you out of trouble," and his hypotheses about how he may have caused the postoperative jaundice by injuring the common bile duct with sutures.

A third aspect of careful thought about decisions is awareness of how likely various events are. The more likely causes and effects come quickly to the surgeon's mind – for example, the scarred duodenum and the bleeding from the suture line.

Decisions must also take into account how good or bad the results of one's actions can be. Such considerations are evident in this surgeon's script, as when he mentions the possibility of stemming the bleeding through the endoscope and thus saving the patient an operation.

Intuition is an important asset for all of us. Nevertheless, some people have difficulty in acknowledging that we use experience in this way, and some have trouble explaining the basis of their reasoning when someone else asks them to defend their judgements. Therefore, intuition has a bad reputation compared with judgement that comes from careful analysis. However, research [50] has shown that people do worse at some decision tasks when they are asked to perform analysis of the reason for their preference or evaluate the attributes of the different choices.

Intuition is not perfect. Our experience will sometimes mislead us, and we will make mistakes that add to our experience base. Imagine that you're driving around in an unfamiliar city, and you see some landmark, perhaps a petrol pump, and you say, "Oh, now I know where we are," and (despite the protests of your spouse, who has the map) make a faithful turn and wind up on an inescapable entrance to the motorway that you had been trying to avoid. As you face the prospect of being sent miles out of your way, you may lamely offer that the petrol pump you remembered must have been a different one: "I thought I recognised it, but I guess I was wrong."

The fire-fighters that Gary Klein studied were aware that they could misperceive a situation. They were not in a habit of counting on it. The commanders rely on their expectations as one safeguard. If they read a situation correctly, their expectations should match the events. If they are wrong, they can quickly use their experience to notice anomalies. In the example of the vertical fire, the commander walked out of the building as soon as he heard that the fire had spread beyond the second floor. He needed to get another reading about what was happening to the building. The commander who pulled his crew out of the building was so discomfited when his expectations were violated that he took that decision. The decision-makers could formulate clear expectations based on their experiences; so that early in the sequence they could detect that they had gotten it wrong. Fire-fighters are not the only ones who use these cognitive techniques. Here is another surgical case presented to the neurosurgeon.

Diagnostic patterns

Case scenario

A victim of a high-speed motor-vehicle accident is unresponsive to deep pain, with both pupils somewhat dilated and sluggish. The vital signs are blood pressure of 120/80 mm Hg and a pulse of 60. What does your exam consist of? How urgent is the CT scan?

Number one, I am not getting enough information. I obviously want to know if he was ejected or if he hit his head on the steering wheel.

We don't have any other information.

Continued

How long was he down in the road? That's the kind of information that I want to know. I am also not getting a good exam from what I've been told so far. He's unconscious, but I am told he has mildly dilated pupils that are sluggish. That tells me nothing. It still confuses me. You can say that you don't know because he has cataracts or because he's blown away one eye. You can even tell me that you haven't examined him. Any of these answers would be better than telling me that he has bilateral, slightly dilated pupils that are sluggishly reactive. If you can't say whether the pupils react or not, just don't say it. On the basis of that exam, I would say that he is drunk.

Tell us what your neurological exam would be when called to A&E to see this patient.

Level of consciousness.

He is unresponsive to deep pain stimulus.

What about his pupils?

Mildly dilated and sluggish.

Again, I would look to find out exactly what that 'sluggish' means. If they're reactive, he's got a toxic metabolic problem and not a mass problem.

So you would look very carefully to see if they are clinically reactive?

If you have to look at one thing, look at the pupils. With white-matter injury, he could have reactive pupils, but it's more unlikely than likely.

Is unresponsiveness much more likely to be toxic metabolic, even in a high-energy motor-vehicle accident?

It's a tough call. You're putting me on the line. The patient not only has diffuse axonal injury, but he is drunk too. Nobody goes out at 2:00 in the morning and drives 80mph without being drunk. But one of the clinchers is: what's his best motor exam? What's he doing?

He doesn't move a single thing when you stimulate him.

Continued

Not a thing?

No. He is breathing spontaneously.

That doesn't make sense.

He is breathing spontaneously, but he doesn't move a thing when you rub on his sternum.

Then he has to have two injuries. He doesn't move a thing – he's got to have a spinal cord injury.

Do you ever see people deep enough that they won't move a thing?

Yes. But they have fixed and dilated pupils.

Do they always go hand in hand?

Always. A flaccid paralysis with reactive pupils is a spinal fracture. But if he is breathing spontaneously, he has to have his diaphragm intact. That puts it at C3, 4, 5 – keeps your diaphragm alive.

This think-aloud shows how the neurosurgeon intuitively recognised diagnostic patterns in trauma. Of interest here is the power of the neurological exam as a tool for diagnosing and managing central nervous system trauma. The expert neurosurgeon's thinking about this patient is built around it. When instant pattern recognition fails him because the picture is confusing, he goes to this tool to organise his thoughts. He directs his attention explicitly to the three categories: level of consciousness, pupillary response, and best motor exam.

Simultaneously, however, he is engaged in intuitive pattern recognition, identifying the possibility that the man is drunk and focusing on the implications of the neurological exam for the competing hypotheses: mass-occupying lesion, alcohol toxicity, and a combination of the two.

Another feature of the surgeon's thinking is that he uses categorical rules, such as "flaccid paralysis with reactive pupils is a spinal fracture," even though he knows that there can be rare exceptions. He pushes through to the most likely conclusion, to see if it can hold up to scrutiny, before going back to consider the rare exceptions.

You may still be wondering: how does pattern recognition work exactly? It is a complex process. It is not like flicking through a photo album in order to identify someone. We don't simply search memory for an exact match. During the pattern matching our brain makes assumptions and fills in gaps based on experience or knowledge. This allows us to function with incomplete information. And, let's face it, if we had to wait until we had all the information, most decisions would be too slow sometimes, with fatal consequences. Thus, pattern recognition allows us to make good judgements without being in possession of all the information. The important aspect is that most of the work our brain does during pattern recognition is unconscious. We either recognise something or we don't. We don't know how we have arrived at the recognition and what assumptions have been made.

One of the factors in pattern recognition being so effective is that the process is unconscious. We are capable of understanding things through unconscious processes that are not processed by the conscious brain. Although we are able to evaluate information carefully by a conscious process, unfortunately it has limited capacity. As you are aware, short-term memory has a limited capacity of seven +/- two units. Hence most of the searching and pattern recognition goes on unconsciously.

In order for us to recognise something, we fill in the gaps in the information we have. Because we do this unconsciously, we are not aware of the assumptions we have made. Pattern recognition works well most of the time. There are some exceptions, though. Sometimes, when we receive unfamiliar inputs that appear familiar, we think we have recognised them, when actually we have not. Thus, by mistake, we match our past experience with the current one when actually it is a mismatch. We have all experienced the embarrassment of approaching a complete stranger we thought we recognised. The second problem occurs when we are filling the gaps. Since gaps are filled by an unconscious process, we are not aware of how they have been filled. This makes it difficult for us to adjust our thinking or to make changes in pattern recognition. The more understanding we have about the pattern, the smaller the gaps would be and the lower the chance of mistakes.

When we have the relevant experience, we can assess the situation and decide what to do faster. But when we are new to a situation, we can get it wrong. You only have to watch someone who has never played tennis before – standing in the wrong place, swinging at the wrong time and sending the ball to the wrong part of the court – to realise this. We are all capable of mistakes when faced with unfamiliar conditions. However, inexpert tennis players know they are getting it wrong. They have ample data to tell them that their technique is not working. Much of the time, however, it is not so easy for us to see that our judgement is flawed. In fact, we are most at risk of making bad decisions when we have enough experience to believe that we are right. It is the expert tennis player fooled by an unfamiliar change in altitude, ball composition, court surface, or racquet length that we are most interested in. Because our pattern recognition depends on input-matching and gap-filling processes that work well when we have sufficient relevant experience, we can be caught out, because we think we have sufficient experience in situations when in fact we do not. We can believe we are being wise when we are being foolish. This propensity for error is easy to observe in fast and speedy decisions. But does it have the same consequences in decisions that often take a longer time, group thinking, analysis and debate? The answer is that it can and does, even for experts. We are all at risk of erroneous pattern recognition, even for those decisions that we take most care over. As a result, we need to identify when it may occur and put in place some defences to reduce the possibility that we will make flawed judgements.

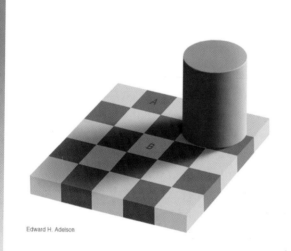

Edward H. Adelson

Reprinted with permission from Finkelstein S, et al [51].

Our ability to create our own reality is illustrated by the figure of black and white checks [51, 52]. One is marked A and another B. Which square do you think has darker shading? Your judgement should tell you, if it is the same as ours, that square A has the darker shading. However, we are wrong. Both squares have the same shading. You will find this hard to believe because your pattern-recognition process is telling you that B is lighter.

In reality, both A and B have the same shading. If you want to prove this to yourself, then photocopy this page, cut out the two squares and put them side by side, or fold the page so that both squares are next to each other.

So what is happening? Why has pattern recognition let us down? It is because our pattern-recognition processes are not about identifying exact matches, but are rather about using similarities and knowledge to arrive at interpretations. We recognise the black-and-white chessboard. We note that square B is lighter than the square next to it. Hence, we conclude that B is a white square. Since B is a white square and A is a black square, B must be lighter than A. So we see B as lighter than A. In scientific terms, we have created our own reality. We then find it difficult to see that the two squares have the same shading, because the process of creating our own reality involves making a change in our store memories. The experience indents itself on our neurones and influences how we integrate situations in the future. Hence, we are partly influenced by previous imprints from seeing other chessboards and partly influenced by the initial imprint from seeing this picture. The combination makes it difficult for us to see that the two squares have the same shading.

Key points

♦ Intuitive thinking is a sacred gift; we need to appreciate the gift and nurture it.

♦ Surgeons rely on intuitive thinking in their day-to-day professional life although they may not appreciate it.

♦ Pattern recognition forms a significant componant of intuitive thinking.

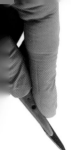

Chapter 6

How surgeons think

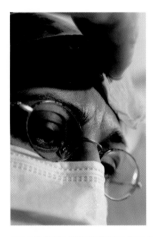

Charles Abernathy, a surgeon, and Robert Hamm, a psychologist, both from the USA, have studied surgeons' intuitive thinking [53]. They invited trainees and experienced surgeons to take part in 'think aloud' sessions on surgical cases. They presented clinical scenarios and transcribed the surgeons' responses in a book of 'surgical scripts'. The psychologist made comments on surgeons' thinking so that others could understand how surgeons with varied experience think. Here is the abridged version of some cases. (I am grateful to the authors for their permission to use the material.)

Case scenario 1 – How experience works

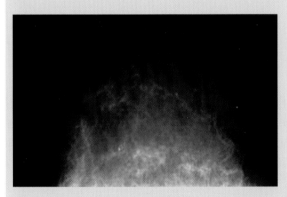

A 41-year-old woman with a large mass in the upper quadrant of her breast has a negative mammogram, and an ultrasound reveals that the mass is non-cystic. You are examining her. What are you going to do?

If this is an asymmetric mass on physical examination and I'm convinced that there is an abnormality, then it's important to know other things, such as family history. But you still come down to the basic question: to biopsy or not to biopsy? And if there's any question in my mind, I biopsy.

Continued

Do you do a needle biopsy or an open biopsy?

If it's a diffuse nondescript mass, I do an open biopsy, because I don't want a sampling error.

Comments

The surgeon's decision depended on experience. In a climate in which the doctor is blamed if a cancer is considered and missed, a biopsy is done if there is any doubt. It can be anticipated that less-experienced doctors will biopsy more often. The expert, then, uses his knowledge primarily to decide which of the lumps not to biopsy.

What happens in the mind as one gains experience? The experts' judgements about which lumps not to biopsy are based on their own experience and on knowledge transmitted from others.

Experience

The experts themselves have felt the breast lumps and seen the subsequent findings on biopsies. They have made a correlation between the two, so that when the lump in a new patient feels like earlier lumps that were not cancerous, they can judge it as unlikely to be cancer. Managing these sensory impressions challenges one's ability to co-ordinate information. In fact, experimental studies have shown that people do not learn very well from outcome feedback: observing a series of events in which an initial appearance (such as the feel of a lump) is followed by an outcome (such as the result of a biopsy) does not allow them to learn what is associated with what. They learn more quickly if you tell them the associations.

Knowledge from others

The other way to learn about the connection between the feel of breast masses and the probability of cancer (and hence about the usefulness of biopsy if other tests are negative) is through verbal communication with others. For this, of course, one must know the vocabulary for describing how the breast feels – e.g. the size, firmness, symmetry, or diffuseness of the mass (the same terms that one may use in learning from one's own experience). And someone has to have previously discovered the valid relations.

Case scenario 2 – Surgeons' reliance on visual and tactile imagery

You just opened the abdomen of a 62-year-old woman with gallstones on whom you are operating for presumed chronic cholecystitis. On exploring the abdomen you feel a 4-5cm vague mass in the head of the pancreas.

I need to determine if it is rock hard or if it is just pancreatitis. There are stones in the gallbladder, so the mass could be a common duct stone. I would feel now for any enlarged nodes in the region, and then re-explore the abdomen to see if there are tiny metastases in the liver on the peritoneal surface or anywhere else.

You don't feel any metastases.

I would do kocherisation of the duodenum to get my fingers underneath the mass, with my thumb on top and my fingers underneath the duodenum and behind the pancreas.

It is definitely a mass, but it is poorly defined.

I see two choices for biopsy: insertion of a Travenol needle either directly into the pancreas or right through both walls of the duodenum from a lateral approach. I would try to avoid piercing the common duct. I would look at the common duct now and dissect the material over it. I would not take out the gallbladder until I knew the diameter of the common duct, because I may need the gallbladder to divert the biliary tract if the common duct is small.

The common duct looks to be about 1cm in diameter, just on the borderline of being enlarged.

I would try to get a cholangiogram in some way. I don't think I would want to get it through the cystic duct, because I would need to keep everything intact in case I need the gallbladder. Because I am sure now that there is a mass in the pancreas, although I'm still not sure if it is pancreatitis or not,

Continued

I would stick a Travenol needle, one stick at a time, into the head of the pancreas – into the hardest part of the mass – to see if I can get a diagnosis. I would freeze each stick one at a time. I want to see if the results are negative. Having done that, I would try to do a cholangiogram through the gallbladder, realising that it is going to take a lot of dye to fill the gallbladder. I would have to try to position things so that the gallbladder dye doesn't obscure the distal duct. I would stick a needle in the gallbladder in an area I probably would use for an anastomosis.

The cholangiogram shows what seems to be a tumour at the distal duct. The frozen section shows an adenocarcinoma of the pancreas.

I know the cholangiogram is not 100% reliable. Now I would begin to ease my finger down along the posterior surface of the tumour, which I have now dissected out, to see if it is stuck to the portal vein. I would also isolate the superior mesenteric vein inferior to the pancreas and the superior mesenteric artery and begin to dissect out these areas. If they are free of tumour, I would now know that the tumour is probably resectable.

Comments

In this think-aloud the surgeon attempts to present visual and tactile imagery as he focuses on the details of the manipulations. The description focuses on what the organs are imagined to feel like ("rock hard" pancreas), and on actions that would be done in exploring (feeling for nodes) or operating (positioning things so that the gallbladder dye doesn't obscure the distal duct).

Although the surgeon is simply talking about organs and does not seem to invoke any higher reasoning, a great deal of knowledge and thinking are still involved here. Strategies reflect sophisticated considerations and experience, for example, "I would not take out the gallbladder until I knew the diameter of the common duct, because I may need the gallbladder to divert the biliary tract if the common duct is small."

In the next think-aloud, the case was presented to surgeons at three different levels: an SHO, a registrar, and a consultant.

Case scenario 3 – Experience changes the thinking

A 57-year-old man comes to the emergency department. He has had two days of left lower-quadrant abdominal pain and what he thought was a low-grade fever. The WBC is 12.5, his temperature is 38.5°C, and the left lower quadrant is tender. You admit him to hospital. What are your thoughts about the patient?

SHO

I have already examined him and taken a history. I would get an X-ray of the abdomen, acquire a stool sample to see if he is bleeding, and make sure that he is stable.

Registrar

I would start with his history to see whether he has had any similar attacks before, any abdominal pain, any abdominal surgery or symptoms that he hasn't been able to describe well, like diarrhoea or a change in bowel habits. I would examine him to get an idea of how tender he is and do a rectal examination to make sure he is not bleeding from below. In a 57-year-old man, especially one with abdominal pain on his left side, you wonder about diverticulitis. I would want an X-ray of the abdomen, to see if he has a normal gas pattern or if there is any perforation; anything that needs taking him to the operation theatre urgently. Beyond that, I would admit him and put him on IV antibiotics to make sure he gets fluid and is well hydrated. You may have to operate acutely.

Consultant surgeon

The things that crossed my mind first are: perforated diverticulitis, cancer, ischaemic colitis – a kind of broad differential diagnosis. The first step I think is general resuscitation more than anything else. I would assess fluids, urine output, and acid-base balance. Then an early decision needs to be made about whether or not he should go to the operation theatre. Peritoneal findings would shift me towards wanting to explore him if I felt he was clinically stable. At that point, I would be inclined to get a CT scan of the abdomen.

Continued

On day one you get a CT scan. His temperature is still 38.5°C, and he still has the same abdominal pain and tenderness. The CT scan shows oedema of the left colon wall.

SHO

That's all? If I have not taken blood cultures, I would do that. I would probably at least consider an endoscopy.

Registrar

The CT scan tells me that the problem is the colon. It could still be diverticulitis, ischaemia, colitis, diarrhoea, or anything like that.

Consultant

At this point, I would think that the overall picture is consistent with diverticular disease or ischaemic colitis. I would be interested in his physical examination at this point.

His fever mounts to between 38.5°C and 39°C every day. On day five, his blood count rises to 16,000. He is still tender in the left lower quadrant.

SHO

I would probably consider repeating the CT examination. I would check the abdominal examination and make sure that it has not changed.

Registrar

You could scope him to look for anything that would sway you from operating, but, at that point, you are still concerned that he has an abscess and needs an operation.

Consultant

At this point, I think that the patient has failed conservative therapy.

Comments

Remarkable here are the differences between the surgeons' responses to the same case, which are a result of their levels of experience. The SHO has a rudimentary response, naming a few tests and emphasising the patient's stability. He shows little evidence of understanding what is, or could be, going on and mentions no specific hypotheses about possible causes of the left lower-quadrant pain. In particular, he seems to have no conception of what may require an operation.

The SHO demonstrates a general understanding of the case. But he does not know what to expect, or what the likely findings of the examination and history would have been. If given more time to think, he could have produced a respectable list of possible causes and appropriate responses. But this information was not available to his mind immediately on hearing the case. His knowledge is not yet organised to provide instant recognition.

The registrar shows a comprehensive and structured response to the case, exceeding not only the SHO but also the consultant in the number of detailed hypotheses and possible tests. The consultant, in contrast, focuses on what is important: the two primary diagnostic candidates, the need for resuscitation, and the need to consider whether an immediate operation is required. The registrar reaches the same points eventually but includes ideas that the consultant did not consider worth mentioning. Because any hypothesis can trigger a test, the generation of numerous hypotheses increases the chances of iatrogenic harm. In addition, it has been observed that residents at intermediate levels of training may actually do worse than either novices or experts. The consultant organises his thoughts around the following key decision: "An early decision needs to be made as to whether or not he should go to the theatre." The registrar's thoughts, on the other hand, dwell longer within the generic structure of the diagnostic patient encounter: "What conditions do I suspect? What tests would I do? What questions would I ask?"

With experience, the expert has developed an organised body of knowledge that is both complete and automatically accessible. The registrar shows an intermediate developmental stage in this process: knowledge that is well structured and rich but does not yet rapidly and automatically focus on the most important aspects of the situation. The automaticity comes with many repeated responses to similar situations, and the correctness of the automatic response depends on whether the resident has engaged in deliberate consideration many times along the way.

We see evidence of such deliberation around the decision whether to go to theatre after the developments (such as increased WBC) on the fifth day. At this point, the consultant immediately concludes that conservative therapy has failed and that it is time to go to theatre. The registrar reaches the same conclusion, but also questions himself to check whether that decision is correct. Such checking, done habitually, keeps knowledge and practice correct; at the same time, they are slowly becoming automatic through repeated use.

Given this context, it would be silly for a registrar to try to emulate the expert by making momentous decisions quickly and without checking. Such shooting from the hip would probably produce errors at an unacceptable rate. Of course, individuals vary in their degrees of cautiousness: some will obsessively review their first responses for years after the accurate response has become automatic, whereas others have to be told to slow down and to think it through.

Case scenario 4* - Decision involves thinking with analysis, or with intuition

A 65-year-old woman presents with a two-week history of weakness in the right hand and leg. What would you do?

SHO

I would do a complete examination to see if anything else is obvious. Are there any other cranial nerve defects? Is anything else in her neurological exam missing?

What else would you do?

SHO

After completing the examination, I would find out if she has any risks for stroke, artery disease in her neck, or heart disease. I would make sure she does not have diabetes – that's it.

Continued

This case discussion is taken from a time where the surgical decisions would be different compared to today. Now it is recommended that people with a mini stroke should have surgery as soon as possible; the decision-making has changed radically. This case has been included here to highlight the fact that although clinical facts may have changed over the years, the process of thinking has remained the same.

Registrar

First I would get a history and physical examination. I would assess whether any associated neurological changes suggest a stroke, a stroke in evolution, or an impending stroke. Has this been a continuous process, or did the symptoms appear suddenly? I would get a CT scan of her head as well. I would work up her carotid arteries, first with a Duplex ultrasound, then with a CT scan. I would proceed on the basis of those findings. I would also do a complete vascular examination, looking for other potential vascular problems. I have found by experience that people with a vascular problem in one area often have vascular problems in other areas. I would also feel her aorta, check her distal pulses, and so forth. In addition, I would look at her history for possible cardiac problems.

Consultant surgeon

History and physical wise, I would want to know if she had ever had any episodes like that before, or any other neurological events, or any other indication of arrhythmias, or atherosclerotic problems. If she was clean from that aspect, I would probably order a CT scan of her head – presuming there are no other tricks to the neurological examination – just to exclude tumour or subdural or other space-occupying lesions. Once I was satisfied with that, I would probably run her by the non-invasive laboratory, but regardless of these results she would probably get a CT carotid angiogram.

Duplex ultrasound reveals a high-grade stenosis of the left internal carotid artery (ICA) and an occlusion of the right ICA. CT carotid arteriography demonstrates an occlusion of the right ICA and 95% stenosis of the left ICA with an irregular plaque. What would you do?

SHO

Has she been improving over these two weeks? ... What would I do...? I would find out if she has coronary artery disease. She is symptomatic from

Continued

an injury, from a low-flow state, because she doesn't have any symptoms on the other side. I think we have to try an endarterectomy.

Registrar

Because of the patient's recent history, I have to state again that I would get a CT scan to look for evidence of a recent stroke. That would make a significant difference in terms of the staging, the specific timing of the operative intervention. If there is no evidence of a recent stroke, I would proceed with addressing the plaque, the stenosis.

Wait a second! Her symptoms are right-sided and it is left-sided stenosis. So I shunt her, regardless of the stump pressures.

Consultant

I would counsel her that there is an extremely high risk of further events and that they will be potentially catastrophic. I would review in my mind the options, such as an external carotid, internal carotid bypass, which is out of favour, but in situations like this it is a thought. I would reject that option and fix her left carotid artery. Using general anaesthesia and a shunt, I would do a left carotid endarterectomy.

The patient was admitted to the hospital. A CT scan of the head demonstrated a small sub-acute infarct of the left cerebral hemisphere. She was treated with IV heparin and admitted to the ICU. Her neurological examination partially resolved over the next 12 hours. Now what would you do?

SHO

You can continue to treat with heparin and see if resolution continues, but you have to solve the problem. At some point, you still have to go into her carotid.

Continued

Registrar

In that case, these symptoms have been going on for two weeks. I would forgo an operation at this point, with demonstration of a recent infarct. I would forgo an operation and assume that her symptoms are secondary to the stroke, not due to an ongoing decreased blood supply or embolic plaque upstream. I would continue to treat her with heparin and do the operation in approximately eight weeks' time.

Consultant

This addresses one point that I did not address: the timing of the left carotid endarterectomy. If the CT scan reveals an infarct, which is unusual, I would try to get specific information from the CT scan or from MRI about the acuteness. These studies may be able to tell you that, depending on the amount of oedema around that infarct. But I think that the patient is in great danger. I would not worry about converting the white infarct to a red infarct. She is two weeks past the initial event and she has improved. Sometime in the next week or two after I have given her aspirin and so forth, I would fix the carotid artery.

Comments

The surgeons' thoughts about this case reveal several aspects of surgical intuition that are related to the question of how long to wait before operating.

The SHO had a common-sense response to the case, a quick intuitive take that she could not follow through on because of lack of knowledge.

The timing of the operation

The timing of the carotid endarterectomy was the key in this case. The consultant surgeon has identified the ultimate struggle between the studies in the literature that show patients to be worse off with early surgery, versus the high chance of a stroke for every week that nothing is done.

As the surgeon who presented the case explained, the patient was actually operated on at the time (her second day in hospital) rather than waiting. This violated the standard practice that after a recent stroke one should wait before operating on the carotids in order to avoid "turning a white infarct red". He had done the operation early after careful consideration and reading, figuring that although the probability of intra-operative disaster was 10%, the probability of an equivalent disaster during a wait of several weeks was 20%.

The registrar, following the standard cautious practice, said that he would wait eight weeks on top of the two weeks the patient had already waited before coming to the hospital. The consultant said he would wait another one or two weeks, which would lessen the time during which a disaster could happen. This is an example of the surgeon's intuitive judgement: without explicitly analysing the situation, he came up with a delay period that reflects the various factors – balancing the danger of "turning the white infarct red" by operating immediately against the danger that another white infarct may happen during the delay. Typical of the processes usually involved in judgement, his immediate intuitive response represents an average of the conflicting considerations: he chose to wait a short period, a compromise between waiting a long period and not waiting at all. His thinking on this issue was an intuitive, integrative judgement rather than the result of a simple rule (like the registrar) or a careful analysis (like the surgeon who presented the problem).

Case scenario 5 – With experience, surgeons rely on more specific maxims

A 65-year-old obese man, who is a known alcoholic, presents to A&E with a two-year history of severe epigastric abdominal pain. His BP is 200/110 mm Hg, pulse is 110 per minute, and his stool is positive for occult blood.

FY1

I am very concerned about his abdominal pain and his tachycardia. I am worried that he has intra-abdominal bleeding of some kind. I would like to know how long he has had the abdominal pain.

Continued

SHO

First of all, you have to instigate resuscitation. Then you begin your investigation to determine the nature of his abdominal pain. Basic laboratory tests should be ordered, chest X-ray, KUB. Specifically, you entertain diagnoses such as duodenal ulcer, perforated or not, some sort of gastric problem, problems associated with the history of alcoholism and potentially a history of blood clot.

Registrar

I first thought of an ulcer disease or some other alcohol-related duodenal or gastric process, but, in the back of my mind, I think that I need to rule out something separate from the alcohol disease, like an abdominal aortic aneurysm, especially in view of the epigastric pain. With the positive occult blood in the stool, I think of an ulcer and something going along with that. I want to know if he has been vomiting and what that would show. I would like to get more information about related symptoms.

Consultant surgeon

Obese, alcoholic male with epigastric pain and positive occult blood in stool. I am going to start IVs and get some baseline laboratory data and a CT scan. I certainly want a full blood count to see whether he has lost a significant amount of blood. Maybe, baseline liver function tests and an X-ray of his chest. I am thinking, epigastric pain in an alcoholic male: gastritis, perforated ulcer. Biliary tract is unlikely.

The patient has an Hb of 9, an arterial pO_2 of 7.25, a pCO_2 of 80, and a base deficit of 10. The abdominal ultrasound in A&E is non-diagnostic because of obesity. His ECG shows sinus tachycardia, his LFTs are within normal range, his BP is 100 mm Hg and his pulse is 120.

FY1

The patient is acidotic and so far that is the only abnormal test result I know about. His blood pressure is dropping, and I am still very concerned about the abdominal bleeding.

Continued

SHO

We have not established a diagnosis yet. The patient is acidotic. His BP continues to drop and he is becoming more tachycardic despite the resuscitation. Therefore, I would consider some sort of intra-abdominal catastrophe. A few critical pieces of information are still missing.

Registrar

It sounds like a perforated duodenal ulcer. Since he is acidotic, he is going into shock.

Consultant

I would do an abdominal examination to see if he is tender anywhere. I would put in an NG tube to see if we are really dealing with upper GI bleeding. Pain plus a drop in BP might mean a ruptured aneurysm. CT could help. I don't think an upper GI endoscopy is going to help.

A CT scan is done, which confirms a 6cm abdominal aortic aneurysm.

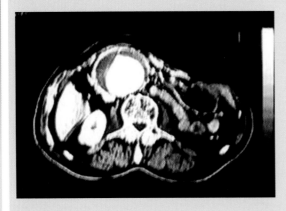

FY1

He needs an operation.

Continued

SHO

He need to be taken to theatre.

Registrar

We are going to have to operate.

Consultant

I don't think we have much time to mess around. We are heading towards the operation theatre.

Comments

This set of think-alouds, by surgeons at four different levels of experience, makes it very easy to see the progression in the ideas that the surgeons bring to the case. We can see differences in what the surgeons recognise and in the strategies they use.

The ideas that come to mind become both more detailed and more focused as one gains experience. The FY1, who saw abdominal pain and high blood pressure, worried about intra-abdominal bleeding. This, of course, is correct, but non-specific. The others show more specific ideas. They look for particular observations or test results and have more specific explanations for the patient's symptoms. The first-year trainee is still trying to figure out what to notice, whereas the more experienced residents usually notice the right facts but still have to figure out what to do with them.

Both the registrar and the consultant surgeon considered the possibility of an abdominal aortic aneurysm before it was reported in the CT scan results. They mentioned it at different times. The registrar mentioned it after the first description of the patient as part of his broad initial response. The consultant mentioned it after receiving the laboratory tests and hearing of the sudden drop in blood pressure. For the registrar, it was a general rule: "If an alcoholic presents with belly pain, rule out abdominal aortic aneurysm before assuming ulcer." For the consultant, it was a more specific recognition: "Pain plus drop in blood pressure may mean ruptured aneurysm." The difference between the two is a sign of 'tuning' one's knowledge. The consultant's mind works more efficiently, applying hypotheses when they are most likely to be needed, and not bothering to consider them explicitly when there is not yet sufficient reason to do so.

When you don't have a well-tuned script that enables you to recognise automatically the key features of the situation, to identify the important hypotheses, and to respond appropriately, you have to figure out the situation logically. In this kind of problem-solving, rules of thumb can be helpful. As one gains experience, the rules become more specific, as befits more specific knowledge.

Thus, the FY1 guides his thinking with a very general rule: "Pay attention to what brought the patient in." This rule orients him to the need to find out all the facts, yet reminds him not to become distracted by aspects of the patient's history that are unrelated to the present illness. The registrar also uses a rule: "Don't get fooled by the most obvious hypothesis," which reminds him to keep other hypotheses in mind and to look for opportunities to rule them out. Even though this general rule helped him to state the correct hypothesis of abdominal aortic aneurysm early in his thinking, the observation of the drop in blood pressure did not return his attention to it. At that point the consultant recognised the correct hypothesis, although he had not explicitly put it on his initial list.

Key points

♦ Cognitive science can reveal how surgeons' thinking changes with experience.

♦ Metacognition, i.e. thinking about thinking, is an established process to improve performance. The case scenarios depicted above show how metacognition can be applied to surgery.

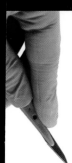

Chapter 7

Smart surgeons – sharp decisions
How do they do it?

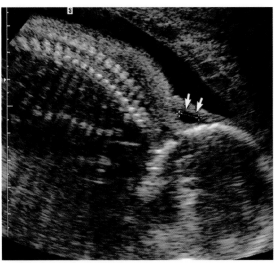

Reproduced with permission from the Radiological Society of North America, © 1999 [55].

A foetus was diagnosed as having a large cystic hygroma [47, 54]. The sonography showed that the hygroma had grown inside the neck, wrapping around the trachea. There was a risk of the infant being unable to breathe after the delivery. A Caesarean section was scheduled for the following day. During the delivery, the doctor in charge was going to determine if the baby was able to breathe on his own. If the baby could not, he was planning to intubate. If he was unable to intubate, he planned to do a tracheostomy, which would be a difficult procedure as the cystic hygroma was filling the space between the trachea and the skin. Upon delivery, the infant gave a cry, suggesting patent trachea. But after the cry the infant could not even grunt. The nurse suctioned the infant's mouth and placed him in front of the doctor.

The doctor remembered an earlier situation, when he had been called in to operate on a young man who had run his motorbike into a strand of barbed wire. The wire had jumbled the victim's neck tissue into sausage-like chunks. On that occasion, the paramedic had inserted an endotracheal tube. When the doctor wondered how this was done, the paramedic later explained that he stuck the tube where he saw bubbles. Bubbles meant air coming out.

So, in the delivery room, the doctor looked into the mouth of the infant for bubbles. All he saw was a mass of yellow cysts, completely obscuring the vocal cords. No bubbles. What the doctor did was place his palm on the infant's chest and press down, to force the last bit of air out of the infant's lungs. The doctor saw a few tiny bubbles of saliva between some of the cysts and inserted the tube into that area. The infant quickly changed colour. The procedure had worked.

This case involved high-pressure decision-making. The doctor did not have any established procedure for inserting the endotracheal tube into the infant in such a situation. He recalled an analogous case – and a far-fetched one at that. It was about someone else's action, not his own. The key point of similarity was discovering the air passage in an obscured throat. And even the analogy was not sufficient. There were no bubbles. The doctor had to invent his own way to produce bubbles.

This kind of skilful decision-making is impressive because, after the fact, the solution seems obvious, yet we know that, without any guidance, many people would miss the solution. They would not even know that an answer was possible. They might have looked into the infant's mouth, see the mass of cysts, and abandon the idea of intubation, immediately resorting to tracheostomy.

Just as we are impressed when someone with expertise seems to know just what to do in a difficult situation, we are also impressed when someone invents a new idea or technique on the spot. This creativity is the product of intuitive thinking. Experts use this kind of intuitive thinking to create a new course of action. They also use intuition to notice something that is not so obvious to pick up but may cause problems at a later stage. They are also able to figure out what is causing the difficulty.

Expert thinking

Whenever a senior surgeon makes a difficult decision that nobody else thought of, we give credit to his experience and say "after all....experience counts....". However, the truth is that it is not just experience that counts. Merely saying that the surgeon used his experience to take the difficult decision is not entirely correct. It is also important to know what kind of thinking was used by the experienced surgeon and to find out how that experience came into play. The general belief is that logical thinking helps the experienced surgeon to make good decisions. However, if we assess the expert surgeon's thought process, you will realise that a significant portion of his thinking is not analytical, but intuitive. Intuitively he is able to size up the clinical situation quickly and imagine how a course of action might be carried out; he also draws upon his experience by suggesting parallels between the current situation and something else that he had encountered before. We do not make someone an expert just through training them in analytical thinking. Quite the contrary is true – if we do that, we run the risk of slowing the development of skills.

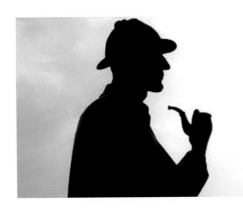

Experts see the clinical situation and match it with their experience. When they start getting initial information, their brain begins to predict what other information they should expect to confirm the pattern. They pick up cues if particular information is missing or there is some information that shouldn't be there. This is one of the most interesting aspects of expert thinking. Not only do they know what they see, they also know what they don't see. You will have come across the stories of Sherlock Holmes – one of Arthur Conan Doyle's stories shows how Sherlock Holmes solved a case using his ability to notice what did not happen. In the story 'Silver Blades', the vital clue was a dog that did not bark at night. The dog usually barked when strangers went by. The fact that the murderer passed the dog in silence meant that the dog recognised him. The absence of a clue helped him to solve the mystery.

Experts appear to have an overall sense of what is happening in a situation. Whereas novices may be confused by all the information, experts see the big picture and appear to be less likely to fall victim to information overload. Also, when we see an expert performing a surgical procedure, he appears smooth and neat. The reason for the smoothness is the detailed knowledge experts have about the procedure. They know not only the bigger picture, but also the smaller steps that constitute the whole procedure.

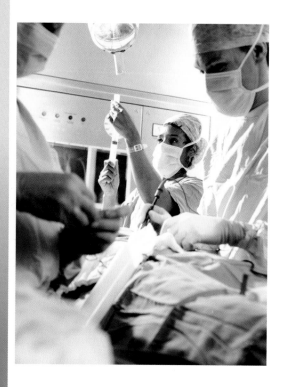

One of the ways of making decisions is to seek additional information. This may seem like a routine activity, but it also requires expertise. A mindless information-gathering strategy is unlikely to be useful. Experienced decision-makers are able to spot circumstances and opportunities in which the information that can be helpful can be readily obtained. Skilled decision-makers may be able to seek information more effectively than novices. This skill in information-seeking would result in a more efficient search for data that clarifies the status of the situation.

Experts in any field can detect differences that novices cannot see, and cannot even force themselves to see. Wine tasters can tell one type of grape from another and even the year of the wine from another. To novices, wines are generic; they all taste the same. If you are just starting to drink wine, no matter how much attention you pay, and how much you swirl the fluid around in your mouth, you don't get it. That is because 'it' is not a fact or an insight. You cannot learn just by being told and you cannot learn all of a sudden. It takes experience, and lots of variety in that experience, to notice the difference.

An important part of expert development is that experts engage in deliberate practice. For them, each opportunity for practice has a goal and evaluation criteria. Mere accumulation of experiences is not sufficient. Experiences need to include feedback that is accurate and timely. In a domain where obtaining timely feedback is not possible, mere accumulation of experience does not result in the growth of expertise. Experts obtain feedback that is accurate and reasonably timely. They enrich their experience by reviewing prior experiences to develop insight and learn lessons from mistakes. In order to perform deliberate practice, people must articulate goals and identify the type of decisions they need to improve.

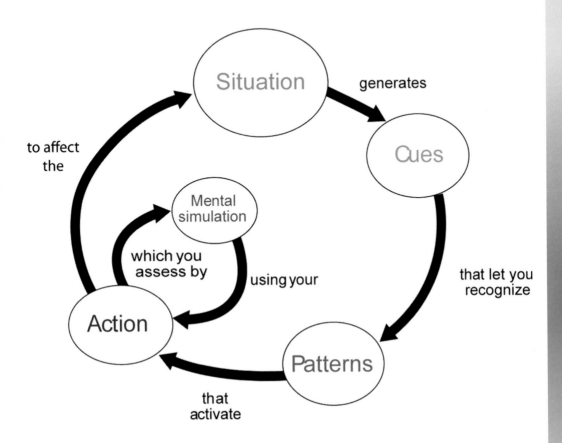

Improving decisions

Since we know that we rely on intuition for good-quality decisions, anybody who is keen to improve their decision-making needs to develop intuition into a reliable tool. We need to treat intuitions as skills that can be acquired like any other skill. Expert surgeons don't just develop good judgement skills, any more than an athlete suddenly has an excellent day on the track. If you are working out for months at fifteen minutes per mile, you are unlikely to sprint seven minutes per mile within a day. This kind of improvement takes effort. Similarly, the kind of judgement that skilled surgeons make also takes work. They have to build up an experience base that lets them accurately size up situations. As with physical exercise, you could get strength by repetitions, but you will get better results if you use an appropriate strategy. In the same way, instead of passively waiting to acquire intuition through routine work, there are methods one can use to speed up the process. One of the methods is to develop the skill of blending intuition with analysis, and another is 'cognitive autopsy' or post-mortem of the decision-making process. For some surgeons, these techniques may be quite obvious. They wonder why such a big deal is made about it. The truth, however, is that it is not obvious to everyone. Even those who understand the importance of intuition do not adopt strategies to achieve good-quality intuition.

Trainees need to make efforts to develop their intuition. The challenge for them is to build intuitive decision-making skills as quickly as possible. We do not get any explicit guidance on developing intuition. As a result, you may flounder, get frustrated, and acquire bad habits and a poor attitude. The higher one goes in the surgical career, the greater the need for intuition. To develop good intuition, one needs to have a collection of various patterns. To develop a range of patterns, we need to get experience. Not every experience is useful for developing intuition. It should be a meaningful experience, an experience that allows us to recognise a pattern and use that pattern as a template for future reference. We think that day-to-day clinical experience is the most meaningful experience. Not necessarily. There are a few problems if you rely solely on clinical experience as a meaningful experience. First of all, getting the satisfactory meaningful experience depends upon chance and circumstances: getting the appropriate job, being supervised by an appropriate surgeon, and so on. Also, the problem with relying on clinical experience is the time required to receive enough experience. It is said that it takes at least ten years to become an expert in any field. With the changes happening in surgical training, surgeons would be expected to develop expertise in a shorter duration. Thus, gaining a meaningful real-life experience is not easy. We need to develop some other ways to seek meaningful experiences. In fact, developing alternative ways to acquire intuitive skills may prove better in some aspects. This is because it would involve 'deliberate practice'. Deliberate practice means not just practising to practice, gathering experience randomly, but practising with specific objectives in mind. Research has shown that meaningful experience and deliberate practice are the most vital ingredients for developing expertise.

Problems of analytical thinking

If we asked anybody what the right way to make an important decision was, we would be told to analyse the problem thoroughly, evaluate all the options, and compare them to see which one was the best. This is a standard method of decision-making and there is something appealing about it. It is based not on whims, but on solid analysis. It is methodical rather than haphazard. It guarantees that you won't miss anything important. It promises you a good decision if you follow the process properly. It allows you to justify your decision to others. It sounds reassuring. Who would not want to be thorough, systematic, and scientific? BUT, there is a problem. The problem is that the whole thing becomes a myth in situations where it matters most. The reality is that this method does not always work well in practice. It works tolerably well on paper, but does not necessarily work in day-to-day clinical life, where decisions are more challenging, situations are more confusing and complex, information is scarce or inconclusive, time is short, and the stakes are high. In these environments, the standard method of decision-making may fall flat.

Nobody would disagree that, without rational analysis, we would not have the exciting growth in science and technology and progress in medicine. Decision trees and cost-benefit analysis can help us make sense of choices, but there are limitations. Just because these methods work in some situations, it does not mean that they work for all practical problems.

Not knowing the problems of this type of thinking, some people take rational thinking to the extreme. They turn out to be hyper-rational. When a person becomes hyper-rational, he attempts to handle all problems, relying only on analytical reasoning. In the initial states, this can be (mis)perceived as a positive sign of critical thinking. Only later do we see an unwillingness to act without a rigid protocol. There is disregard for the needs of individual patients. They even lose a common sense. If the problem is not checked in time, the final stages degenerate into what is called 'paralysis' by analysts. A surgeon just sits on a case, when others would have intervened. To get an idea of how bad the problem of hyper-rationality is, consider two different kinds of ophthalmic diagnoses.

One of the two clinical entities is macular degeneration, in which the fovea and the central zone of the retina are destroyed. The second is retinitis pigmentosa, in which the peripheral vision deteriorates. As we know, the fovea is the only part that is capable of fine discrimination. One may think that macular degeneration could be the worst visual impairment. Retinitis pigmentosa gives the impression of being less devastating than macular degeneration. But the reality is altogether different. Retinitis pigmentosa is a far more disorientating condition than macular degeneration. If you lost all your peripheral vision, you would have a tiny searchlight sweeping endlessly back and forth, trying to locate everything and retain orientation. Without peripheral vision, you would even have trouble sitting quietly and reading, since you need peripheral vision to direct your eye movements. Hyper-rationality is like retinitis pigmentosa, in which we try to do all our thinking with analysis. Rational thinking is like foveal vision using cone cells, which provides us with the ability to make fine discrimination but is not

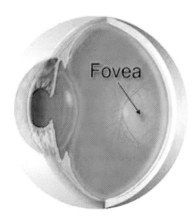

Fovea

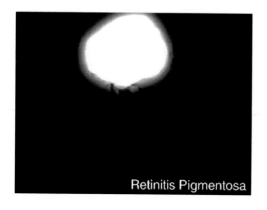

Retinitis Pigmentosa

Macular degeneration

sufficient to maintain orientation, and is irrelevant during night-time. We need peripheral vision to detect where to apply the analysis and calculations.

Although problems with analytical thinking have been mentioned, we need to be aware that intuition cannot solve every problem. Analysis has a proper role as a supporting tool for making intuitive decisions. When time and the necessary information are available, analysis can help uncover cues and patterns. It can sometimes help evaluate a decision. But it cannot replace the intuition that is at the centre of the decision-making process, although that is precisely what some people try to do. We are advised by some to suppress our intuitions, because, according to them, intuitions are inherently biased. One can agree that we shouldn't blindly follow all intuitions, as they can be unreliable and need to be

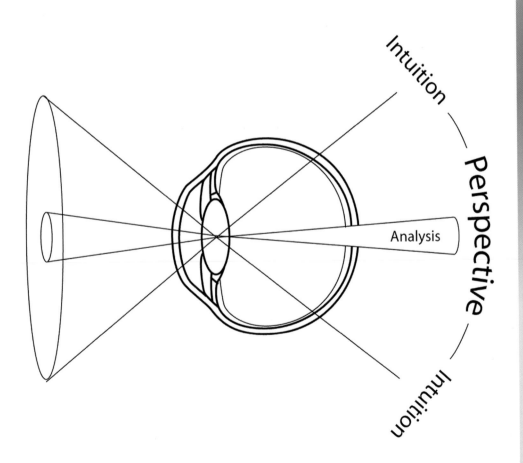

monitored. However, we shouldn't suppress them, either, because they are essential to our optimum decision-making and in some situations can't be replaced by analytical thinking. Thus, our real option is to strengthen our intuitions so that they become more accurate and provide us with better insights. Although intuitions may not always be reliable, they at least guide us in the right direction.

Should we take gut feelings seriously?

Of course we should. Here is an experiment that explains why we should. Neuroscientist Antonio Damasio and his colleagues have published a series of experiments showing that our judgements and emotional reactions to a problem can be expressed even before we have any conscious awareness of the problem [56]. In one experiment subjects were asked to turn over cards from four different decks.

A   B   C   D

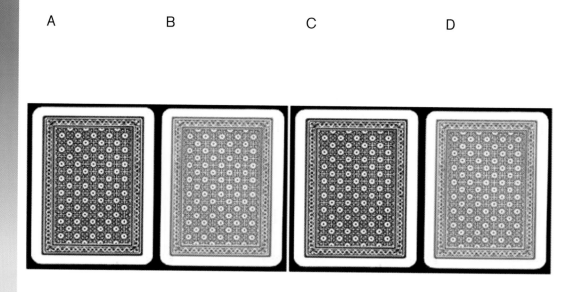

All cards had a monetary value. Each card told the subject whether he had won or lost the money. The subjects were instructed to turn over the card from one of the four decks and to make as much money as possible.

The interesting part of the experiment was that the cards were not distributed evenly or randomly. The scientists had rigged the game. Two of the decks, A and C, were full of cards with high rewards and also high penalties. The other two decks, B and D, by comparison had lesser rewards and lower penalties. If the subjects would have chosen cards only from B and D, at the end they would have far more money than if they would have chosen cards from A and C. The other interesting part of the study was the subjects were monitored by various equipment to observe their emotional reactions, for example, skin electrical conductance tests to observe any anxiety response.

When the subjects started picking the cards, they picked them up randomly, searching for the most lucrative card. However, after drawing about 40-50 cards randomly they started drawing solely from profitable decks. If they were asked at that stage as to why they were selecting only decks B and D, they wouldn't give any explanation. By the time they had turned over 80 cards in total, they were able to explain logically their reasoning behind selecting those decks.

The scientists were not interested in logic, they were interested in emotions. What they found out was that after the subject had drawn only ten cards, his hands got 'nervous' when he approached the negative (A/C) decks. Although the subject had little inkling of which card piles were the most lucrative, his emotions had developed an accurate sense of fear (just as Michael O'Riley developed the same feeling when he saw a missile on the radar in Chapter 5). The intuitive thinking figured out the game first – it found out which decks were dangerous. This intuitive response, which was mixed with emotions, was reflected in physiological parameters. The subjects were neither consciously aware of the physiological response nor were able to verbalise reasoning behind their choice.

The experiment did not stop here. The researchers compared responses of normal subjects to subjects with a specific cerebral pathology. Subjects with a specific cerebral pathology did not show any physiological response. They were unable to figure out the correct strategy as well. Thus, normal subjects were able to gather more money than subjects with cerebral pathology. This experiment is useful for two reasons, first it gives us an explanation as to why we should take gut feelings seriously and, second, it also explains why we call them 'gut feelings'. The term reflects the biological or physiological nature of the thought process.

Thus, you had better take gut feelings seriously, as those feelings are borne out of your experience. Just because they are not conscious, don't dismiss them. There are some limitations of conscious processes. You can only be conscious of one thing at a time. That's why consciousness is a bottleneck. Think about the differences between foveal vision and peripheral vision. If you didn't have peripheral vision, you would have great difficulty in walking, driving and orienting. Peripheral vision can be equated to subconscious thinking. In many situations, conscious analysis of choices does not work. Either there is not enough information, or there is too much information. If there is enough information, it may not be in the right form, or there isn't time to sort through it all. If we couldn't fall back on intuition, we would get stuck much of the time. Intuition lets us stay on cognitive autopilot so that we can focus on other important things at that moment. Intuition enables us to respond to the cues we're barely aware of. Intuition lets us size up the situations in just a few seconds, and also provides early warnings of dangers.

There is some evidence that, when people ignore intuition, the quality of their decisions goes down. People experience this while solving multiple-choice questions. One of the explanations for this phenomenon is that some decisions are made subconsciously, before people even start to perform analysis, and the very act of articulating the factors can make decisions inappropriate. Some research [50] has shown that people do worse at some decision tasks when they are asked to perform analysis of the reason for their preferences, or to evaluate all the attributes of the choices.

Although intuition has its own limitations, it seems that we have made too much of them. Views such as, "intuition is basically untrustworthy," or, "avoid intuition at all costs," are going a bit too far. Going back to the analogy of the visual system, our eyes are not perfect. They have blank spots, focus that creates blurriness, and sometimes require lenses to correct for distortion. Yet we don't reject the information we receive from our eyes. Similarly, just because intuition is fallible, that doesn't mean we can't make good use of it.

Blending analysis and intuition

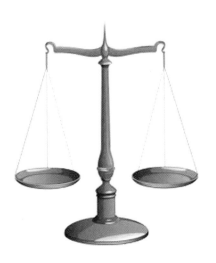

Neither analysis nor intuition alone is sufficient for every decision that needs to be made. Therefore, we need to explore the connection between them, highlighting what can go wrong if we rely excessively on intuition and what can go wrong if we rely too much on analysis. The synthesis between intuition and analysis that seems most effective is when we put intuition in the driver's seat so that it directs our analysis of our circumstances. This way, intuition helps us recognise situations and helps us decide how to react, while analysis verifies our intuitions to make sure they aren't misleading us. Experts in this field recommend starting with intuition, not with analysis. If you begin by analysing a decision, you are inevitably going to suppress your intuition. You are better off starting by getting a sense of your intuitive preference – a gut check of your immediate preference, identifying your intuition before it gets clouded.

Pattern matching provides the initial understanding and recognition of how to react to a particular event, and the mental simulation (imagining how the reaction will play out) provides the deliberate thinking – the analysis – to help us decide if that course of action really would work. A good example of this process is our visual system. The fovea lets us see fine details. When we read, we focus the fovea on the letters. In contrast, peripheral vision is useful for providing the overall perspective that lets us keep ourselves well oriented in space. We need both the fovea and the periphery to carry on our lives. Of the two, the peripheral-vision system is more important. Our intuition functions like our peripheral vision, keeping us oriented and aware of our surroundings. Our analytical abilities, on the other hand, function like foveal vision and enable us to think precisely. We may believe that everything we think and decide comes from our analytical thinking, the conscious and deliberate arguments we construct in our heads, but that is because we are not aware of how our intuition directs our conscious thought processes.

Sometimes we need to rely more on intuition and other times we need to draw on analysis. When the situation keeps changing, when the time pressure is high, or when the aims are fuzzy, you cannot use analysis alone. You have to depend on your intuition. And when you have a lot of experience you can recognise what to do without having to weigh up all the options. In contrast, if you have to find the best option to solve a problem and not just a workable one, you may want to analyse the strengths and weaknesses of each alternative. If you have made a decision but are pressed to justify your choice, the most convincing way is to line up your options and explain why your selection was the wisest choice.

In chess, it is important to find the best move, not just a good one, so players continue to search for the best option. Yet it is also seen that, for the most part, they settle on the first option they had thought of, even after considering many others. It is likely that the first option that you think of while making a decision is the best. Although the results cannot be guaranteed, the observation is backed up by research evidence. Thus, it is important to note your initial impulse when faced with a difficult question. You should think about this option critically. You may discard it after a thought. But, if you ignore it, you would be missing out on some fast and free advice from your subconscious mind. And after thinking through your decision, if you really can't choose between different options, you should probably just go with the first impulse. A warning comes with this advice: do not mix up intuitions with desires. Sometimes, those first impulses are about what we want to happen rather than what is likely to happen.

Cognitive autopsy

Experience is a powerful teacher, but experience by itself is not the most efficient way to learn. The process can often be painful and time consuming. To learn as quickly as possible, we must be more deliberate, more disciplined and more thorough in our approach, in order

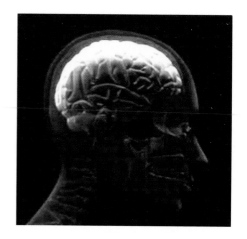

to squeeze as much as possible from each experience. We can treat any experience as an opportunity to learn. There are a number of ways to get feedback about our decisions.

We often give ourselves feedback, too. It is natural for us to mull over our decisions after the fact. We often beat ourselves up over bad decisions and congratulate ourselves for good ones. We 'what if' ourselves. One of the most valuable things we can do is to take this natural tendency and refine and discipline it. But instead of passing judgement about whether it was a good decision or a bad decision, we should focus on understanding the decision process: why we decided what we did and how we made the decision. This type of feedback lets you revise and improve on your intuitions. When you do not have many chances to encounter challenging situations, you have to get the most out of the incidents you have. That means spending time afterwards to see what the incident has taught you. This applies both to real experiences and experiences from other or theoretical discussions. Reflecting on our decisions is particularly useful when we have encountered some difficulty, including cases of failure. Failures grab and hold our attention, and they are loud signals that our mental models were not good enough. Failures hurt and that keeps us from forgetting them.

There are two types of feedback – the first is outcome feedback, which means that the decision-maker is informed about the outcome of his decision. In the case of surgical decisions, it means whether the action resulted in a positive outcome or not.

Case scenario

You are asked to see a critically ill patient with peritonitis. After your assessment you decide to treat the patient conservatively and over the following weeks, the patient recovers from the illness. You consider this as positive feedback to your decision-making.

The other kind of feedback is process feedback, which involves reflecting on how we made decisions and how we could have spotted patterns more quickly.

Case scenario

In the earlier case if you reviewed yourself and the factors that guided you to take the decision of 'wait and watch' – that would be the start of process feedback. If you followed the patient over the course of the next few days and monitored his clinical condition, keeping on track with your decision process that would be considered as process feedback.

Research has shown that we learn significantly better from process feedback and learn much less from outcome feedback.

There is an important point to note here. Poor outcomes are different from poor decisions. The best decision possible given the knowledge available at the time the decision is made can still turn out unhappily. A patient may die unexpectedly despite receiving the correct treatment. A poor decision is one for which we regret the process we used. A person will consider a decision to be poor if the knowledge gained would lead to a different decision if a similar situation arose. Knowing simply that the outcome was unfavourable should not matter. Knowing what you failed to consider would matter.

In addition to feedback, expertise is affected by the opportunity to reflect on experiences. For example, chess masters do not spend all their time playing games against each other. The bulk of their time is spent studying the positions of previous games. During a tournament, a grandmaster will be working against the clock and will not be reflecting on the implications of the game, but afterwards there is time to go over the game record to look for opportunities that were missed, early signs that were not noticed or assessments and assumptions that were incorrect. In this way, an experience (even a single game) can be recycled and reused. In many field settings where there are limited opportunities to gain experience, developing the discipline of reviewing the decision-making process for each incident can be valuable.

We have a system already in place to learn from our experiences and to conduct post-mortems of our decisions: morbidity and mortality meetings. However, we find that the sessions typically get into debates about facts and details and ignore the practical or intuitive decision-making perspective. There is hardly any appropriate discussion taking place on the decision-making process. Instead of brainstorming sessions, they turn into blame-storming sessions. That is like giving people feedback on their driving by listing the cars they hit, without checking out their vision. Ideally, a good session would include a discussion of what was done. But it will also help people to learn about patterns – for instance, when was a problem first spotted, and were there earlier signs that were ignored? How were people interpreting the situation – were there different ideas about what was going on? What happened to make it clear? Could people have obtained more information earlier to reduce uncertainty? Did they wait too long, in the hope that uncertainty would diminish, and should they have acted more quickly to gain an advantage?

Surgeons and uncertainty

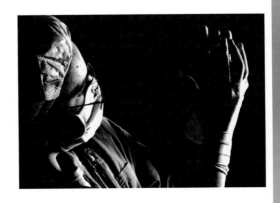

Intuitive thinking is especially helpful when we are dealing with uncertainty. In day-to-day surgical practice, we face uncertainty about many issues. We can be uncertain about the diagnosis. We can be uncertain about what kind of treatment we are going to offer the patient. We may be uncertain about what kind of surgical approach we are going to use for the procedure. Even if we have all the knowledge about available options, we may be uncertain about which is the best option to choose. Frequently we are pushed to make decisions in the face of uncertainty. A senior surgeon once commented "if I am only 40% confident, I think that I need to gather more information. On the other hand, if I am more than 70% confident, I think that I have probably gathered too much information!"

Why do surgeons face clinical uncertainty? We face the uncertainty because you may not be able to obtain sufficient information, some of the vital information may be missing, one of the investigations you have ordered may be unreliable, and the clinical findings and report from the investigations may be giving conflicting information. Thus, there are various factors behind uncertainty. Although all these factors lead to a similar condition – uncertainty, it would be wrong to tuck all these factors under a single label. That way we delay the process of resolving the uncertainty.

Lack of information may be because you have either not received it or are unable to locate it after receiving it. Even if you have located the information, sometimes, it may not be reliable. You may suspect that the information you have is erroneous or outdated. Even if the information may be accurate in actuality, our doubts about its reliability will create uncertainty in our minds. Maybe we have the information and we trust that information, but it appears inconsistent with other information; the examination findings may not be consistent with the history, the investigation reports may not be consistent with each other. To arrive at a diagnosis or treatment decision we may have to skim through a lot of irrelevant information – a kind of 'noise' – but if we are not able to differentiate between relevant and irrelevant information, it adds to our uncertainty. Sometimes we are bombarded with too much data and instructions. In those circumstances we may not have an easy way to recognize the noise. If we are unable to recognize the noise we will not have the confidence to ignore it.

Sometimes we may have all the necessary information which is reliable, consistent and relevant, but we could still be uncertain if we cannot interpret the information and apply it to the clinical context. This happens in very complex cases with multiple comorbidities, where we are unable to recognize a pattern.

It is wise to think about all these aspects of uncertainty due to lack of information, as the cause of missing information will guide you in managing that uncertainty.

Ten strategies surgeons can use to deal with uncertainty

There are various ways to handle uncertainty, and the larger your repertoire of strategies the more flexible and efficient your decision-making can be. We have observed a great deal of (smart!) surgeons with excellent decision-making skills and would like to depict the following range of strategies they employ to deal with uncertainty.

Strategy 1– Delaying

You don't have to offer an immediate decision for every case. In some cases, the crisis that got everyone worked up yesterday turns out not to have been a big deal today. Smart surgeons have a good intuition about what is a real crisis, and so they can safely delay making a move with the understanding that with time the picture will be clearer for appropriate action. I have to raise a cautionary note here. Some surgeons (not so smart!) make the mistake of delaying because they are afraid of making a tough decision under uncertainty. You don't want to lose an opportunity while waiting to get perfect information. This is where intuition is needed, to help you gauge when delay makes sense because the situation is likely to resolve itself or because more information is likely to come in.

Strategy 2 – Obtaining more information

Seeking more information is a common reaction to uncertainty. Sometimes it makes sense, but some surgeons often use information-seeking as a way to buy more time. Nonetheless this strategy is better than the earlier strategy of delaying; at least you are doing something. However, at times, all you are doing is wasting time, especially when there is no point in trying to turn a good plan into a perfect one. If you do need to gather more data, you need to use intuition in doing this. Smart surgeons know when to seek more information and judge whether the information is sufficiently valuable and is likely to arrive in time to make a difference in the ultimate decision.

Strategy 3 – Enhanced monitoring

If you are faced with a major decision and your uncertainty is very high, you may want to change your approach by adopting active or aggressive monitoring of the situation – perhaps calling for more frequent observation or interventional investigations. Some may view this as just seeking more information. However, this is different from obtaining more information as you are not trying to get any specific data. Rather you are monitoring an ongoing situation so you can make your move at just the right moment. Be careful of not overdoing it though – you may end up collecting too much irrelevant information.

Strategy 4 – Filling the blanks

Instead of gathering more data, uncertainty can be reduced by filling the blanks – the missing information – by making assumptions about what the missing information is likely to be. This strategy is a little risky, but this is how smart surgeons prove themselves in difficult situations.

Strategy 5 – Making sense

Once you have gathered the information, you can try to paint a picture of the decision at hand. This strategy goes beyond merely filling in gaps. It is about making sense of the situation – constructing explanations, categorizing situations and also correcting your own. This process of sense-making is very important for intuitive decision-making. 'Sense-making' is the process we use to size up the situation; for example, you are performing a surgical procedure and detect some unexpected anomaly. The surprise we feel signals to us that we need to re-interpret the way we understand the clinical situation. Because of this you would be extra cautious in looking for more cues or findings that might have been missed earlier, but are now seen as important.

We need to make sense of the situations so that we can figure out 'the problem of the day' – the potential trouble spots we have to track closely. We need to make sense of the situation so that we anticipate how a proposed change in a plan is going to play out and what kind of problems might emerge. We also need to make sense of a situation to appreciate what we can realistically achieve.

Strategy 6 – Marching ahead

Despite our preference to have all the necessary information before making a difficult decision, there are times when we have to realize this isn't going to happen. The earlier statement by a senior surgeon, saying that if he does not need to be more than 70% confident for making a decision, reflects his comfort to live with uncertainty. In difficult situations smart surgeons like him press on to implement the plan.

Strategy 7 – Shaking the tree

Sometimes the best way to handle uncertainty is to conduct a pre-emptive strike against it.

You can anticipate a clinical course of a case and make predictions. If you feel that there is a possibility that the situation may get out of control, rather than the situation reaching that stage you take a proactive step. You see this kind of strategy in action when you see a patient during the day and you conclude that the patient would need surgery soon. Currently, the patient is stable and does not necessarily need to be taken to theatre urgently. However, you predict a clinical progression and anticipate that the patient may become critical in the middle of the night. For that reason you decide to take the patient to theatre urgently. To implement this decision, you may have to convince your anaesthetist, nursing staff or management about the urgency, who may not be prepared for an emergency procedure. Thus, in these situations you may need to shake the tree.

Strategy 8 – Making incremental decisions

Instead of deciding all the issues at once, you can make a small change and see if it works. Through these small steps you allow yourself the opportunity to understand the clinical situation, to get feedback and to make improvements. This approach has some drawbacks though. It may signal to others that you are not confident in managing the case. This can affect the morale of the patient, family or your team members. If you are using this strategy, you need to be careful not to be trapped by the 'sunk cost' bias. After you have progressed further in the treatment plan, you may become reluctant to discard the previous efforts by discontinuing the strategy. Your approach to this situation should be to consider a previous plan (which has not worked) as an initial investment – a cost of doing business, not a stake that has to be recouped.

Strategy 9 – Prepare for the worst

Besides considering various other strategies, you also want to plan for the worst possible scenario to make sure that you haven't left yourself vulnerable. Involving other colleagues and adding more resources (either from your side or the patient's side) is a way to make the plan more robust.

Strategy 10 – Embrace the uncertainty

The idea of embracing uncertainty goes beyond simply accepting it – here we are valuing uncertainty for what it adds. Smart surgeons make a virtue of uncertainty, moreover, some thrive on ambiguity. One may wonder if the uncertainty that surgeons face in day-to-day practice is inevitable.

Clearly, the technology available in the future will dramatically increase the information available, yet we cannot be optimistic that increasing information will necessarily reduce uncertainty. It is more likely that the information age will change the challenges posed by uncertainty. Previously, information was missing because no one had collected it; in the future, information will be missing because there is too much information and no one can find the relevant piece. Moreover, improved data collection will likely transform into faster decision cycles. Historically, patients used to stay on the ward for a longer time and we had more time to take decisions. Nowadays a patient's stay on the ward is reduced and we have to take similar decisions in a shorter duration. By way of analogy, when radar was introduced into commercial shipping, it was with the intent of improving safety, so that ships could avoid collisions when visibility was poor. The actual impact was that ships increased their speed, and accident rates stayed constant. Thus, the safety advantage of the radar was neutralised by increased speed of the ships. On the decision front, we expect to find the same thing. Planning cycles will be expedited and plans will be made with the same level of uncertainty as there was before. Moreover, people will expect faster decisions, without the time allowed in the past for thoughtful reflection.

Because uncertainty is inevitable, decisions can never be perfect. Often, we believe that we can improve the decision by collecting more information, but in the process we lose opportunities. Even if you gather information, key pieces may be missing, unreliable, ambiguous, inconsistent, or too complex to interpret, and as a result a decision-maker will be reluctant to act. Because it is impossible to achieve 100% certainty, decision-makers must be able to proceed without having a full understanding of events. Skilled decision-makers appear to know when to wait and when to act. Most importantly, they accept the need to act despite uncertainty.

In 1996, the world chess champion, Gary Kasparov, defeated the IBM chess computer Deep Blue in a six-game match. Observers noted that Deep Blue never adjusted its playing style. It always searched for the best move, even in positions where it knew it was behind. A human would have used intuitive thinking with a strategy that was speculative, rather than marching off to defeat. One of the IBM team members explained that the computer did not have a sense of 'creative desperation' – the sense that drives chess players to search for intuitive decisions, no matter how risky.

How to communicate your intuitions

One of the difficulties in using intuitive decision-making is that you may struggle to express exactly what your intuition is telling you. It isn't enough to make sharp decisions if you can't get them implemented. We experience this problem in two ways; when we try to communicate our reasoning behind the decision to others and also when we struggle to interpret the decision taken by others. We need to find ways to communicate our intentions clearly to others. When others don't understand the reasons behind our instructions, they are ill-equipped to respond to unexpected problems or questions. And when we receive suggestions or views from someone else, we have to reach beyond words to determine what the person is thinking.

One reason that it's hard to share our intuitive skill is that we don't always know what we know. We make judgements all the time based on nothing but a hunch, but rarely do we understand or bother to understand where that hunch came from. You may have hit a brick wall when you asked an expert surgeon "how do you know that?". Either the expert gave you a blank look or gave you a lecture that sounded very intelligent but didn't answer your question.

One strategy to obtain an appropriate answer, for questions like "how do you know ......", is to avoid asking such general questions. Instead of using vague questions if you make a specific inquiry you will receive a better response. You may ask the expert to tell you about another time or another case when a similar type of situation arose. Then one can stretch the incident on the timeline and identify the judgements and decisions that were made. You can ask the expert about the cues and patterns that were available. You can also compare the expert's account with the way you might have approached it. After a good interaction in this manner, experts sometimes express their appreciation because they have learned for themselves what really happened.

In order to explain and share intuitive skills you need to focus on various aspects of decision-making that we have discussed so far, detecting subtle cues and pattern recognition and so on. Surgeons usually apply these strategies without thinking about them. That is why it is hard to describe them to others. And that is why you do better considering a specific incident, because subtle aspects of your experience become more visible.

Final checklist (not again!!!)

We began this book with a 'checklist' and we will also finish with a checklist, although this final checklist is going to be somewhat different as it is an attitude check (list) towards decision-making. After reading this book so far you may have started thinking about your own decision-making process. You may have felt that you have gained some new ideas and tips to give you more understanding. However, to fully benefit from this new information you may have to check your own attitude towards improving decision-making. Here is a list of some unhelpful attitudes people may have to help you identify if you have any of these.

- Experience automatically creates expertise; I don't have to work at it.

This attitude is a justification of negligence. Merely having experience is not enough. True experts take their decision-making skills seriously, setting goals for themselves for areas they would like to improve. To develop expertise you need to receive feedback and you need to make changes accordingly.

- I already have too much on my plate to spend time working in my decision-making skills.

Could it be that you may be feeling overworked because you are going about things the wrong way? If you could follow more efficient decision-making strategies, you may be able to dig yourself out of the hole of overwork. Your current way of doing things may be taking too much time and forcing you to do frequent damage repair.

- You are either born with intuition or you are not.

There is no evidence that intuition is inborn. The type of intuition we have considered depends on experience and pattern recognition, skills people do not automatically have, although there is a case to say that people differ in how open they are to their intuitions.

Finally, you decide

We have less time and fewer chances to achieve expertise in the current surgical climate compared with previous generations. We are faced with additional challenges that further affect our decision-making skills and intuitions. Diminished experience, rapid turnover, little training, increased pace of change, reliance on procedures and protocols – all of these create an unprecedented assault on our intuitions. Why do we tolerate all of these challenges? Because people don't fully understand what intuition is and how it develops. So they are unaware of these barriers and their cumulative effects. The erosion of our intuitive faculty will continue until we take active steps to defend it. The longer we wait to defend our intuitions, the less we will have to defend. We are more than the sum of our software programs and analytical methods, more than the database we can access, more than the procedures we have been asked to memorise. The choice is whether we are going to shrink into these artefacts or expand beyond them. You decide!

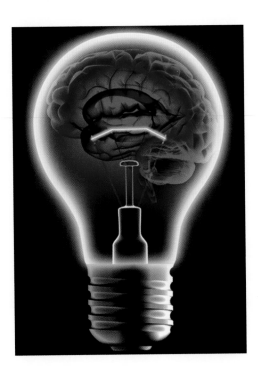

Key points

◆ We do not make someone an expert just through training them in analytical thinking. Quite the contrary is true – if we do that, we run the risk of slowing the development of skills.

◆ Expert surgeons don't just develop good judgement skills, any more than an athlete suddenly has an excellent day on the track.

◆ Meaningful experience and deliberate practice are the most vital ingredients for developing expertise.

◆ Analytical thinking has some weaknesses which affect our decision-making capacity.

◆ A real option is to strengthen our intuitions so that they become more accurate and provide us with better insights. Although intuitions may not always be reliable, they at least guide us in the right direction.

◆ Skilful blending of analysis and intuition offers an optimum strategy.

◆ The synthesis between intuition and analysis seems most effective when we put intuition in the driver's seat so that it directs analysis of our circumstances.

◆ Do not mix up intuitions with desires. Sometimes, first impulses are about what we want to happen rather than what is likely to happen.

◆ Cognitive autopsy offers helpful feedback on decision-making.

◆ Clinical uncertainty is unavoidable; surgeons can adopt strategies to deal with uncertainty.

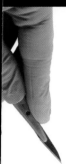

Further reading

1. Hudecek IP. BMJ responses *BMJ* 2009; 338: B517.
2. Quin J. Boxing clever – a global multicenter pilot study of checklist. *BMJ* 2010; 340: C514.
3. National Patient Safety Agency. http://www.npsa.nhs.uk/.
4. Hanks AB, Gawande AG, *et al*. A surgical safety checklist to reduce morbidity and mortality in a global population. *New England Journal of Medicine* 2009; 360: 491-9.
5. Godlee F. Human as hero. *BMJ* 2009; 338: B238.
6. Soar J, Peyton J, *et al*. Surgical safety checklists. *BMJ* 2009; 338: B220.
7. Kohn LT, Corrigan JM, Donaldson MS, Eds. *To Err is Human; Building a Safer Health System*. Washington DC: National Academy Press, 2000: 220.
8. Flin R, O'Connor P, Crichton M. *Introduction, Safety at the Sharp End*. Ashgate Publishing, 2009: 3.
9. Helmreich RL, Merritt AC. *Culture at Work; National, Organizational and Professional Influences*. Aldershot, UK; Ashgate Publishing, 1998.
10. Irita K, Kawashima Y, Morita K, Seo N, Iwao Y, Tsuzaki K, Makita K, Kobayashi Y, Sanuki M, Sawa T, Obara H, Omura A. Critical events in the operating room among 1,440,776 patients with ASA PS 1 grade one for elective surgery. *Japanese Journal of Anesthesiology* 2005; 54(8): 939-48.
11. Yule S, Flin R, Patterson-Brown S, Maran N. Non-technical skills for surgeons in the operating room: a review of the literature. *Surgery* 2006; 139(2): 140-9.
12. Dekker SWA, Hugh TB. Laparoscopic bile duct injury: understanding the psychology and heuristics of the error. *ANZ J Surgery* 2008; 78: 1109-14.
13. Cuschieri A. Nature of human error: implications for surgical practice. *Annals of Surgery* 2006; 244(5): 642-8.
14. Wilson JA. Practical Guide to Risk Management in Surgery: Developing and Planning Healthcare Risk Resources International. Royal College of Surgeons symposium, 1999.
15. Kwaan MR, Studdart D, Zinner MJ, Gawande A. Incidence, patterns and prevention of wrong site surgery. *Archives of Surgery* 2006; 141: 353-8.

16. Allison RE. *Global Disasters.* Upper saddle river, NJ: Prentice-Hall, 1993: 11-2.

17. Gawande A. *Complications: A Surgeon's Notes On An Imperfect Science.* Picador, 2003.

18. Way LW, Stewart L, Gantert W, Liu K, Lee CM, Whang K, Hunter JG. Causes and prevention of laparoscopic bile duct injuries: analysis of 252 cases from a human factors and cognitive psychology perspective. *Annals of Surgery* 2003; 237: 460-9.

19. Hugh T. New strategies to prevent laparoscopic bile duct injuries – surgeons can learn from pilots. *Surgery* 2002; 132: 826-34.

20. Hall JC, Ellis C, Handorf J. Cognition and surgeon. *British Journal of Surgery* 2003; 90: 10-6.

21. Groopman J. Surgery and satisfaction. *How Doctors Think.* New York: Houghton Mifflin Harcourt Publishing Company, 2007: 156.

22. Meakins JL. Evidence-based surgery. *Surgical Clinics of North America* 2006; 86(1): 1-16.

23. Larsson J, Weibull H, Larsson B. Analysis of the decision-making process leading to appendectomy: a grounded theory study. *Scandinavian Journal of Psychology* 2004; 45: 449-54.

24. Quality assurance programme, Swedish Surgical Society, 1995.

25. Marteau T, Sowden A, Armstrong D. Implementing research finding in practice: beyond the information deficit model. In: *Getting Research Findings into Practice.* Haines A, Donald A, Eds. London: BMJ publications, 1998: 32-42.

26. Greenhalgh T, Robert G, McFarlane F, Bate P. Diffusion of innovations in service organisations: systematic review and recommendations for future research. *Milbank Q* 2004; 82: 581-629.

27. LeBoeuf RA, Shafir EB. Decision making. *In: The Cambridge Handbook of Thinking and Reasoning.* Holyoak KJ, Morrison RG, Eds. Cambridge: Cambridge University Press, 2005: 244-6.

28. Kahneman D, Tversky A. Choices, values and frames. *American Psychologist* 1984; 39: 341-50.

29. Mcneil BJ, Pauker S, Sox H, Tversky A. On the elicitation of preferences on alternative therapy. *New England Journal of Medicine* 1982; 306: 1259-62.

30. Sassi F, McKee M. Do clinicians always maximise patient outcomes? A conjoint analysis of references for carotid artery testing. *Journal of Health Service Research Policy* 2008; 13(2): 61-5.

31. Patkin M, Isabell L. Ergonomics, engineering and surgery of endo-surgical dissection. *Journal of the Royal College of Surgeons of Edinburgh* 1995; 40: 120-32.

32. Tversky A, Kahneman D. Availability: a heuristic for judging frequency and probability. In: *Judgment under Uncertainty: Heuristics and Biases.* Kahneman D, Slovic P, Tversky A, Eds. Cambridge: Cambridge University Press, 1982: 163-78.

33. Potchen EJ, Cooper TG, Sierra AE, Aben GR, Potchen MJ, Potter MG, Siebert JE. Measuring performance in chest radiography. *Radiology* 2000; 217(2): 456-9.

34. Redelmeier DA, Koehler DJ, Liberman V, Tversky A. Probability judgement in medicine; discounting unspecified possibilities. *Medical Decision Making* 1995; 15(3): 227-30.

35. Tversky B. Visuospatial reasoning. In: *The Cambridge Handbook of Thinking and Reasoning.* Holyoak KJ, Morrison RG, Eds. Cambridge: Cambridge University Press, 2005: 209-32.

36. Woods DD. The alarm problem and directed attention in dynamic fault management. *Ergonomics* 1995; 38: 2371-93.

37. Potchen EJ, Sierra AE. Value judgements in diagnostic radiology: how do we decide? *Radiology* 1981; 138(2): 501-4.

38. Fischhoff B, Beyth R. I knew it would happen – remembered probabilities of once – future things. In: *Organisational Behavior and Human Performance* 1975; 13(1): 1-16.

39. Arkes HR, Wortman RL, Saville PD, Harkness AR. Hindsight bias among physicians weighing the likelihood of diagnoses. *Journal of Applied Psychology* 1981; 66: 252-4.

40. Chapman GB, Elstein AS. Cognitive processes and biases in medical decision-making. In: *Decision-making in Health Care.* Chapman GB, Sonnenberg FA. Cambridge: Cambridge University Press, 2000: 196.

41. Ritov I, Baron J. Reluctance to vaccinate: omission bias and ambiguity. *Journal Behavioural Decision-making* 1989; 3(4): 263-77.

42. Redelmeier DA, Shafir E. Medical decision-making in situations that offer multiple alternatives. *The Journal of the American Medical Association* 1995; 273(4): 302-5.

43. Croskerry P. Achieving quality in clinical decision making: cognitive strategies and detection of bias. *Academic Emergency Medicine* 2002; 9(11): 1184-1204.

44. Shanafelt TD, Balch C, Bechamps G, Russell T, Dyrbye L, *et al.* Burnout and career satisfaction among American Surgeons. *Annals of Surgery* 2009; 250(3): 463-71.

45. Hastie R, Dawes RM. *Rational Choice in an Uncertain World.* Thousand Oaks, CA: Sage, 2001: 36-45.

46. Croskerry P. The importance of cognitive errors in diagnosis and strategies to minimise them. *Academic Medicine* 2003; 78(8): 775-9.

47. Klein G. *Sources of Power.* MIT Press, 1998: 35.

48. Benner P, Tanner C. How expert nurses use intuition. *Am J Nursing* 1987; 87: 23-31.

49. Klein G. *Power of Intuition.* MIT Press, 1998: 13.

50. Wilson TD, Schooler JW. Thinking too much; introspection can reduce the quality of preferences and decisions. *Journal of Personality and Social Psychology* 1991; 60: 181-92.

51. Finkelstein S, Whitehead J, Campbell A. *Think Again: Why Good Leaders Make Bad Decisions and How to Keep It From Happening to You.* Harvard Business Press, 2009.

52. http://web.mit.edu/persci/people/adelson/checkershadow_illusion.htm.

53. Abernathy CM, Hamm RM. *Surgical Scripts.* Hanley & Belfus Inc., 1994.

54. Berlinger NT. Vital signs: The breath of life. *Discover* 1996; 17(3): 102-4B.

55. Mernagh JR, Mohide PT, Lappalainen RE, Fedoryshin JG. US assessment of the fetal head and neck: a state-of-the-art pictoral review. *RadioGraphics* 1999; 19: S229-41.

56. Bechara A, Damasio H, Tranel D, Damasio AR. Deciding advantageously before knowing the advantageous strategy. *Science* 1997; 275: 133-7.